# I'M SO effing HUNGRY

# I'M SO
## effing
# HUNGRY

Why We Crave What We Crave—
and What to Do About It

AMY SHAH, MD

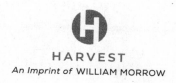

HARVEST
*An Imprint of* WILLIAM MORROW

I'M SO EFFING HUNGRY. Copyright © 2023 by Amy Shah, MD. All rights reserved. Printed in the United States of America. No part of this book may be used or reproduced in any manner whatsoever without written permission except in the case of brief quotations embodied in critical articles and reviews. For information, address HarperCollins Publishers, 195 Broadway, New York, NY 10007.

HarperCollins books may be purchased for educational, business, or sales promotional use. For information, please email the Special Markets Department at SPsales@harpercollins.com.

FIRST EDITION

Library of Congress Cataloging-in-Publication Data has been applied for.

ISBN 978-0-358-71691-4

22 23 24 25 26 LBC 5 4 3 2 1

To my wonderful husband, Akshay, and my two children, Jaden and Lara, without whom this book would have been completed one year earlier. Jokes aside, I owe them everything and more. Thank you for being my rocks. And to my readers—I am nothing without you. I have so much gratitude for you.

# Contents

# Introduction

*It's Not Your Fault*

I ONCE CAUGHT AN EPISODE OF *Sex and the City* that made me laugh, cringe, and feel sad all at the same time. Miranda Hobbes—the brilliant, hard-working, efficient, and articulate corporate lawyer—was standing in her kitchen.

Miranda picked up a small piece of chocolate cake and ate it, but then decided to toss the rest of the cake into the garbage can, presumably to stop herself from finishing it off. But wait—she then plucked another piece of the cake right out of the trash can and devoured it. Disgusted, she squirted liquid dishwashing detergent over the trashed cake so there was no way to wash the cake off, much less eat it.

Amusing? Yes. Gross? Kinda. Unusual? No!

Honestly, it is very normal to crave certain foods, and these cravings are not always the result of the disordered eating seen in this fictional example. I've talked to, and worked with, thousands of people from all walks of life and from all over the world who deal with hunger issues and cravings. They make three-o'clock runs to the coffeehouse for a latte and sweet treat, open the fridge to satisfy midnight cravings, eat off their kids' plates, love sugary foods, plan cheat days, and all the while go on and off diets. In every city they've ever lived, they can give you directions from any part of it to the nearest convenience store, fast food joint, donut shop, or deli.

And why?

Because they feel famished all the time, even after finishing off a delicious meal. Or they simply crave sweet, salty, or crunchy stuff constantly. Or they're lonely or stressed out, and to comfort themselves, they cave into cravings. Some are just plain addicted to food, especially sugar, and feel very out of control with food in their eating habits.

Many of these women (myself included) have suffered through never-ending, harmful cycles of weight loss and weight gain. They've tried diet clubs, low-carb, keto, paleo, vegan, and other flavor-of-the-month diets so many times that they've lost count. They've stressed over all this and have struggled with their poor relationship with food.

Let me tell you a story about my 37-year-old patient Monica, who like the fictional Miranda was an attorney with a successful practice. She restricted her food intake during the week but went overboard on the weekends with lots of wine and late-night, carb-filled meals. She would eat a full meal, only to continue eating second and third helpings. During a vacation to Colombia one year, she was served a dinner of fresh breaded shrimp on board a boat—a local specialty. As she drank more wine, she ate more until she was stuffed. Yet she couldn't stop—and even went for a third helping, snuck in after everyone else was asleep.

On a deeper psychological side, Monica was depressed by this behavior and had developed so much anxiety over food that she couldn't eat anything without guilt. She felt out of control when it came to her appetite and eating, and she didn't know how much food was enough.

Monica asked me, "Am I crazy for doing this?" Of course, I assured her that she was not and that she was not at all alone, and that her story is all too common these days.

For many women like Monica, hunger has become their great enemy, and they're constantly fighting it. The battle steals their self-confidence, piles on guilt (and pounds), and makes their spirits ache. This fight has owned them for so long that freedom from it seems elusive.

You get the picture.

Maybe you're in it.

And you're wondering: Why am I so effing hungry?

## THE REAL REASONS FOR HUNGER

So many people (like the old me) needlessly go through life suffering because of their relationship with food and constant need to give in to cravings They feel like food cravings have a strong hold over their lives. They walk around all day, thinking about their next meal. They feel beaten down by their lack of willpower to resist food. Nobody wants to go through life like this, but it happens despite their best intentions—far more often than you might realize.

Does any of this sound familiar?

If so, I've got the best possible news for you: Constant hunger and cravings are not your fault! Seriously, I repeat, it's not your fault.

They are NOT caused by a result of what you DO. Nor are they a sign of weakness or a lack of strength. And they have little to do with willpower. Willpower, self-restraint, discipline—none of that effing matters in this case. So repeat after me: "It's not my fault."

Okay, so I know you're wondering—"If it's not my fault, what exactly is the problem?"

There are not one but three big problems at work. I will elaborate a bit more in this introduction and explain in much greater detail throughout the book, but here's the short version. The first problem has to do with a societal response to food that has been engineered by food manufacturers to be highly palatable and addictive.

The second is a psychological response, often brought on by moods or emotions. Emotional triggers to eat include stress, loneliness, habit, boredom, or anger, as well as more enjoyable feelings like happiness and celebration. (Food companies capitalize on these issues, too.)

The third is a physiological response—controlled by your brain and your gut and of which you are unaware—that causes your hunger and satiety (fullness) signals to stop working as they should. True hunger, of course, is mostly a physiological need for nutrients to fuel your body. Just like your car requires gas to function, your body needs food and nutrients to survive and thrive. Once your tank is empty, you must refill it.

So, when you find yourself constantly hungry, craving certain foods, and not able to stop eating—these are the main reasons why this happens.

This is largely information no one has told you about before, at least not the food and diet industries. And probably not even your doctor. Doctors will blame you for your hunger and cravings because they don't understand the physiology or the neuroscience themselves—these topics are not taught in medical school.

For decades, we've been brainwashed to believe that if someone has a weight problem it's because they eat too much. They need to consume fewer calories than they burn—slashing calories and eliminating foods is the answer. And if you do this, you too can look like Gwyneth Paltrow! Not true—and a total myth. (No offense, Gwyneth!)

In fact, in medical school, doctors are taught this myth—and we're taught that to solve the issue, people just have to stop eating so much. But it turns out it's not that easy. Being overweight and gaining excess weight are not simply a matter of calories in and calories out. There's so much more, including the involvement of hormones and the neuroscience of hunger and appetite. These factors, however, are not adequately covered in medical school, unfortunately.

And don't think for a moment you'll always be a prisoner of your cravings—without a solution. You can do something about this and I'm going to give you the solution in this book. The program I share in these pages will naturally tame out-of-control hunger and cravings, help you trust your hunger signals, stop dieting, and free you from negative feelings associated with food and eating.

This book and the 5-step plan evolved from my experiences studying nutrition, becoming a doctor, working with patients, and researching little-known facts about the gut, brain, emotions, and hunger. It was developed to help the thousands of people like you with whom I've worked over the past few years and who have struggled with hunger, cravings, food anxiety and guilt, weight ups and downs—and have even been known to walk twenty blocks for their favorite dessert. Happily, using this plan and its steps, my patients have escaped the angst of being hungry all the time. The same success can happen to you! (You'll read more of my patients' stories later in this book, and I know they will inspire you and give you hope.)

Now for some background.

## UNRAVELING THE
## MYSTERIES OF HUNGER

Before I became a double-board-certified doctor of medicine (internal medicine and allergy/immunology), I obtained a bachelor's degree in nutrition at Cornell University's Division of Nutritional Sciences, which offers one of the country's top-notch programs.

Nutrition was a topic that had always fascinated me. In high school, I became worried after my grandmother was diagnosed with type 2 diabetes—a disease my grandfather had died from when he was only 60. Not only that, my dad and his four brothers had all been diagnosed with diabetes in their early thirties. One of my uncles is a cardiologist who once reminded us over a carb-filled family dinner that no one in our family lived past the age of 60.

Since moving to the U.S. at age 5, I had noticed that my parents' dietary habits started to veer from eating the vegetarian-based meals of our Indian culture—lots of vegetables, roti, and other traditional foods—toward eating more of the processed foods so prevalent in a Western diet. Although they still enjoyed our traditional cuisine, they began to eat pizza, fast food, and nachos a few nights a week and drank a lot of cola. Doritos became their favorite snack. I knew this behavior was largely responsible for their diabetes and had certainly worsened it. I wanted to figure out how to curb these eating habits and prevent my family and other families from having to deal with diabetes and its possible consequences.

What also terrified me was that diabetes doesn't just affect someone in the short term. It is a leading cause of death because it triggers the onset of cardiovascular disease, kidney and nerve problems, and many other serious issues.

These weren't just things that happen to other people, either. They were happening right in my own family. So I decided to take an active role in my father's health care by monitoring his diet and nutrition and trying different diets with him—high fat, low carb, vegan, paleo, Ayurveda (a natural system of medicine that originated in India more than three thousand years ago that I learned growing up in my family's culture), among others. When I got involved, my father was game to make changes, and I was proud of his attitude and motivation.

Eventually, we landed on a plan that worked—and worked wonders. Over a two-year period, my father went from using 50 units of insulin to fewer than 20, lost 30 pounds, and received consistent reports of improved health from his doctor. And he no longer craved sugary, processed foods.

Over the years, I refined this plan based on my education and experience as a doctor. Now it forms the blueprint of the programs I tailor for my patients and clients and led to my writing my first book, *I'm So Effing Tired,* in 2021.

With this new book—*I'm So Effing Hungry*—I cover brand-new territory. Different hormones. Different insights into nutrition. Different plan. Plus, I present cutting-edge science about what goes on inside the body to control hunger, appetite, and cravings. Hunger is a completely different beast than fatigue, and in this book you'll learn some amazing facts about why you're so effing hungry and what to do about it.

My mission is to revolutionize the way people eat. To change the way they think about hunger and nutrition. To help them handle hunger and cravings—and break free from the tyranny of diets and battles with food. This program can give you the tools to handle all the "hunger" you have in life (i.e., "hunger" for good relationships, more purpose, bigger impact). I've seen my program work for women all over the world. And it will work for you, too.

I'm thankful I started on this path by studying nutrition first. It taught me about food science, the role of nutrients, what happens to your body when you eat different foods, and the various diseases associated with nutritional deficiencies. Not many doctors have this kind of background.

When I was a nutrition student at Cornell, I attended nutritional conferences and seminars to augment my knowledge. It was at these events that I became aware of a strange and alarming disconnect.

I remember with crystal clarity the first conference I went to. Held at the Hynes Convention Center in Boston, the conference was littered with booths decorated with huge, bold, and colorful banners and where freebies, pens, and other knickknacks were being given out. I entered the center, frazzled and sweating from trying to find a parking space and walking around in ill-fitting high heels to try to fit in. I was young and inexperienced but I was there to absorb. After registering, I was handed a huge canvas bag filled with samples and pamphlets from food giants like Nestlé, General Mills, and Kraft.

Educational sessions were sponsored by different companies, particularly big-name cereal companies. One seminar covered how gluten was being falsely accused of causing gastrointestinal troubles. I was surprised. Whenever I ate gluten, my stomach hurt, I lost energy, and I got bloated. A lot of people are sensitive to gluten, and I'm one of them—so I was mystified by hearing gluten being presented in such a positive light—and without acknowledgment of those who had a sensitivity.

There was also a session covering the China Study—a huge research project about the health benefits of a vegan diet—in which the presenter discussed the link between eating meat and developing cancer. As a lifelong vegetarian, I was fascinated by that session. But I was MORE shocked to see so much processed meat served at the luncheon right after this seminar!

Overall, I just couldn't believe there was so much blatant promotion of processed food over real food at a convention where nutrition was the topic. No wonder so many people were dealing with weight gain, obesity, diabetes, and other food-related illnesses—many medical professionals and practitioners didn't even have a basic familiarity with good nutrition.

Those experiences really opened my eyes. We were (and are) being so duped! These conventions, which normalize or even encourage the consumption of processed food and dismiss health trends that focus on food sensitivities, are part of the societal connection to hunger that I mentioned earlier.

I went on to medical school, first at the Albert Einstein College of Medicine in New York City, followed by a residency at Harvard Medical School's Beth Israel Deaconess Medical Center in Boston. Three years later, I was accepted into the Columbia Presbyterian Hospital/Columbia University immunology program.

While I was in medical school, I was taught everything a doctor-to-be needed to know about anatomy, physiology, disease, and treatments. But I don't remember learning much about nutrition or preventive medicine. What little I did learn comprised about 15 percent of my nutritional knowledge.

After many years of school and training, I started my private practice, thrilled to put all my training to work. But deep down, I knew that my special training and expertise would be mostly wasted in the Western model of medicine, with its emphasis on treating symptoms rather than finding the root causes of illness and preventing them. Western medicine has some strengths in addition to its weaknesses, for sure, and it is great in an emergency or when surgery is needed. But it often fails to support illness prevention and the self-healing processes that go on inside the body.

I was determined to change the way I practiced medicine to impact more people.

While all of my education has been enormously important and formed a tremendous foundation, I decided to teach and practice in a way that was different, using my South Asian upbringing and my special in-depth training in nutrition and immunology to treat people successfully. I'm named as a medical doctor on my diplomas, but I consider myself a practitioner of integrative medicine as well. This means that I focus on healing through nutrition, wellness, and lifestyle.

# PSYCHOBIOTICS, HUNGER, CRAVINGS—AND YOU

Since the publication of my first book, *I'm So Effing Tired*—which offers a proven plan for overcoming the issue of fatigue in women—I've been studying the forces behind excessive hunger and food cravings.

As I mentioned, I was motivated to explore this topic because so many of my patients as well as other women were telling my how constantly hungry they were and that they prayed that the next day would be different. Their urges for different types of food—sugary, salty, crunchy, and all of the above—were strong and real. Some could open a bag of potato chips and eat every chip in a single setting or finish off a quart (or more) of ice cream for dessert.

But there's a deeply personal side to my exploration into hunger and cravings: my own life. When I was in my early thirties, I felt like my life was blowing up. I was a wife and mom with two toddlers at home. I was building my medical practice. I was spending a large share of my free time with toxic people who were bad for my mental health. I was so worn out that I could not focus and get control over my schedule and daily life tasks. Then—partly because of my go-go-go hurried lifestyle—I was in a horrific car accident in which I almost lost my life. In the midst of the recovery and healing process, there were too many balls to juggle in my life, and I felt like I couldn't stop the stress and chaos.

My only coping mechanism for the stress was to eat—and not the right foods. Those choices only intensified my cravings. I was sleep-deprived too, which made me even hungrier.

Then my amazing husband stepped in and insisted that I needed to create more boundaries in my life to rein in and reduce the stress. I listened to him. We agreed that we both needed a major health overhaul, my husband as much as me.

We committed to making some sweeping adjustments in our health and nutrition. We changed the way we ate—emphasizing natural, whole foods most of the time. (I taught myself to stop self-medicating with food, using the techniques you'll learn in this book.) We exercised more gently—and especially outdoors in nature. We did more yoga and meditated. We stopped engaging with people who were bringing us down. Little by little, my whole life started to change. I finally made it to the other side, and I was a new person.

So yes, I get it. You are overwhelmed just like I was overwhelmed. You are right to question why this is happening to you. I can help you, not just because I'm a medical doctor, but because I have been there, and I know what it takes to empower yourself again.

When it comes to cravings, we women may have it worse. Published in *The Yale Journal of Biology and Medicine* in 2016, one study pointed out that women find it harder to regulate food cravings compared to men. Only 20 percent of women who reported cravings indicated that it was "easy" for them to resist cravings, as compared to 50 percent of men.

As I realized this was a problem without a clear-cut solution, I just happened to be reading about a relatively new concept in alternative medicine called psychobiotics. This term refers to the live microbes living in the gut that have been shown to impact the brain and the nervous system. Key processes in your body (including hunger, weight, even your mood) are tightly regulated most of the time by these live bacteria. Scientists have known about this relationship for awhile, but it was practically dismissed because it was thought to be unimportant. Now we know better. Studies of psychobiotics have begun to unveil the impact of this relationship on almost every part of the body.

Here's where it gets interesting. These microbes know how to make message-sending neurotransmitters (normally manufactured by the brain) all on their own. They don't have brains, of course, but they use neurotransmitters like the chemicals dopamine and serotonin to communicate with each other, just like brain cells do. They may also be communicating with us as well and have quite a bit of influence over how we feel, think, and react.

One of the most fascinating new discoveries, reported in such journals as *Nutrients* and *Trends in Neuroscience*, is that microbes are using these chemicals to control our appetite and make us crave certain foods. So when these microscopic critters get hungry for sugar and other foods, you get cravings for the same foods! This is a big reason why you're so effing hungry. And if you're deficient in certain gut bacteria, you may be more likely to feel famished all the time, crave various foods—and suffer from mood disorders—including depression (which doesn't help cravings in the least). Hunger and cravings are much more nuanced than modern Western medicine would have you believe.

I've devoted a whole chapter to psychobiotics, so I don't want to give away the plot here. But the big takeaway is that psychobiotics are one of the main causes of hunger and cravings, not your weakness or lack of discipline. It's not even your fault if you're overweight, either. You just might be eating foods that affect the diversity of microbes in your gut, and that imbalance is making your body store fat—this is all part of psychobiotics too.

## THE FOOD INDUSTRY AND HUNGER

Remember my story about the food industry and its sponsorship of nutrition conferences? Well, it's that very same industry that is formulating and selling foods designed to be addictive and irresistible so that we keep coming back for more, despite the consequences.

Food manufacturers actually hire engineers to manipulate combinations of sugar and fat or fat and salt to elicit the ultimate pleasure response in people, as measured by electrodes attached to brain areas that light up when these combinations are eaten. In the processed food industry this response is referred to as the bliss point.

Here's something wild: food manufacturers have also altered the distribution of fat goblets in some foods to affect absorption rate (this is known as the mouth feel), changed the physical shape of salt so it hits taste buds harder and faster (this is known as the flavor burst), and added condensed chemicals that are known to trigger intense pleasure responses.

The combined effect of these factors is that we're now bombarded with highly palatable foods that are combinations of sugar and fat (like ice cream, cookies, and cakes) or fat and salt (such as nuts, potato chips, and French fries) that trigger us to eat more of them.

And if we're feeling emotional? Watch out, because emotions are a further trigger to overeat. But even emotional eating is not your fault. The part of your brain—the midbrain—that craves social interaction is the same part of the brain that hungers for food. So if you feel lonely, you're apt to get hungry, even if you've just finished a big meal!

Reaching for sugary foods under any circumstances is a bad deal. Because these foods are easy to digest, they break down rapidly and flood the digestive system all at once. There, they eff up hormones involved in hunger and satiety. A key hunger hormone—ghrelin—is stimulated, which makes you feel hungrier as you eat and after you eat. This process shuts down the production of leptin, the I'm-full hormone. Besides driving up your cravings for more of this processed food, the net effect of this mess makes you want to eat even after you're full.

I know, this sounds like mad scientist stuff, but it's happening all around us, without our knowledge, and one of the simplest examples is concocted every day at your local McDonald's. Have you ever thought that a Coke from McDonald's tastes so much better than one from anywhere else? Here's why: McDonald's buys cola syrup from Coca-Cola—but at a McDonald's restaurant, less carbonated water is added in a prechilled mix ratio to the syrup than at other places that serve Coke from a fountain. That's one of the main reasons why a Coke at McDonald's is sweeter and just generally tastier than a cup of the stuff from anywhere else.

As for diet sodas, I've watched multiple TikToks that have gone viral, rating the best diet cola. I always know which brand is going to win!

What's more, the straws at McDonald's are slightly wider than typical straws, so more of that liquid goodness hits your tastebuds all at once. At least with straws, bigger really IS better. If you can't seem to stop sipping long after you've washed down your burger and fries, now you know why.

See what's happening? These companies are taking addictive substances and making them more addictive! No wonder we're so effing hungry. I've got more eye-opening stories about the food industry to share with you later in the book that will make you think twice about hitting the drive-through or opening a bag of chips.

## THIS IS NOT A DIET BOOK

In my practice, I work with a lot of people who want to lose weight, and they want it off by next Friday. Being at a healthy weight is a great goal, and you don't need a medical degree to know that it cuts your risk factors for cardiovascular disease, high blood pressure, type 2 diabetes, certain cancers, and other scary illnesses.

In today's world, however, people are overly fixated on losing weight and they try to follow diets that take a restrictive, quick-fix approach to weight control. Most are simply not sustainable. You grit your teeth and try to stick with the diet in question for a couple of weeks or for thirty days, until you can't anymore. Then you go back to your normal way of eating because you miss lasagna or ice cream and back come the pounds, with interest, and the cycle repeats.

Your gut bacteria enter the picture once again, too. They do a lot more than assist with good digestion. They produce chemicals that make you hungry. Some types of bacteria chop food into tiny pieces that get digested, add calories to your body, and thus tend to pack on pounds. If your gut has more of those kinds of bacteria—which happens when eating too much processed food—it is tougher to lose weight.

After being a doctor for almost twenty years, I can also tell you this: most diets are a product of a diet industry that has taught us to deny and dismiss our hunger cues and rely instead on lists of food to eat, when, and in what portions. This industry would also have us believe that controlling our weight is about personal responsibility, discipline, and willpower, and that hunger is bad.

Tell that to my patient Cyndie, who at 250 pounds was dealing with diabetes and liver and heart problems until she stopped dieting and learned to listen to her body and eat real food. She not only lost quite a bit of weight, she also broke free from the vicious cycle of warring with her own body about hunger, cravings, and food. The whole culture around dieting has also created guilt and other negative feelings about food and our bodies. It's sad and I know you can relate.

Here's a startling stat: as of 2019, the U.S. weight-loss market is booming and the diet industry has grown to a record $72 billion. This growth is expected to reach a mind-blowing $253 billion in the next five years, according to AXcess news.

If all these diets worked, then why is this growth trending upward so fast?

You've probably heard the phrase "follow the money," right? When we follow this money, it's easy to see why the diet industry—ironically and tragically—wants to keep us fat and sick. No one makes money when people are at peace with their bodies.

Still, many dieters believe that to shed pounds, and even to maintain their weight loss, they have to stay hungry all the time. I'm here to tell you that you don't.

You see, food is the necessity of life. We can't live without it, but we need to make peace with that fact. There are different and delicious varieties of foods we should include in our diet on a regular basis for better body functioning like nutrient intake, healthy digestion, increased muscle mass, hydration, adequate energy, and so on. It is impossible to live without food!

Further, our lives do not center on diets and calorie counting—they're a rich tapestry of experiences that fulfill us in many different ways. A more holistic approach to better health starts with the way we talk (and think) about eating and hunger as it affects our health.

In fact, true physical hunger—the kind that is a brief signal to eat—is necessary for survival. It tells us exactly how much to eat to keep at a healthy weight for our bodies. Most of us have not experienced true hunger since we were toddlers. But after you get back in touch with it, you will instinctually know how much to eat, and you will not gain weight.

So I'm not giving you a diet here, and I'm not giving you any diet rules. The only rule here is that there are no rules.

What I'm giving you is the power of choice when it comes to food. You must eat in order to live, and your state of health depends on making better, more nutritious food choices more often. Doing so will give you freedom and peace.

I'm also offering you the knowledge and power to make friends with food, not feel deprived, and eat according to what your body tells you to eat so you can make important permanent changes—the kind you can live with the rest of your life. In doing so, you'll liberate yourself from constant hunger and cravings—and the self-defeating cycle of weight loss and weight regain.

## What about Eating Disorders?

This book is not about eating disorders—which are complex mental health problems that must be addressed by medical and psychological intervention. Most have a variety of symptoms, including severe restriction of food or purging behaviors like vomiting or over-exercising. Eating disorders are not only caused by issues with hunger or cravings, but also by genetics, personality traits like perfectionism, and a perceived pressure to be thin.

If you suspect you or someone you love suffers from an eating disorder, please seek the help of a qualified mental health counselor.

## MY PLAN AND HOW TO USE IT

I've taken everything I've learned from years of research and experience and wrapped it up in this easy-to-understand book. This book summarizes all the science, debunks mainstream myths about hunger, and provides you with actionable, science-based strategies you can employ immediately to manage false hunger and cravings.

This book will bring you face-to-face with the truth about why you're so effing hungry, why it's not your fault, and what to do about it. With every piece of this information, you'll be equipped to:

- Discover little-known yet powerful facts about certain foods and nutrients that will manage your hunger and cravings—effortlessly and automatically.
- Escape the forbidden food diet mentality and learn to make a friend of food.
- Rewire your brain and manipulate certain hunger/satiety neurons so that you naturally reach for healthier options—no willpower required.
- Learn to read the patterns of hunger versus cravings.
- Leverage the powerful connection involved in what you eat, your gut health, your brain and neurons, and your mood.
- Stop fighting the scale and make peace with your body.
- Bring your body back into healthy balance with behavioral and lifestyle strategies that refresh your brain, and stop decades-old dieting patterns.

So—how are you and I going to accomplish all this?

With a 5-prong approach.

Step 1: Replenish. I don't focus on what you remove from your diet (unlike every other plan out there). I show you how to add in daily targeted nutrients, called the Super Six and found in foods you eat every day, that will automatically curb your hunger, control cravings, and normalize those hungry gut microbes. Not only that, these foods boost your metabolism, quench the flames of inflammation, lift your mood, equip your body to fend off illness—and more. I'll show you how to incorporate these foods into your diet with a simple and flexible meal plan that includes some delicious and satisfying recipes.

Step 2: Rewire. As I've said, we've been hijacked by the food and diet industries to crave foods and processed junk. With this step, I show you how to reclaim what these forces have stolen from you by rewiring your brain to stop the addiction/hunger pathways.

Step 3: Reset. Hunger is regulated in part by our circadian rhythm, a vital internal clock that governs the sleep–wake cycle and repeats about every twenty-four hours. When this cycle is off—usually due to stress and the hecticness of modern lifestyles—you can get ravenously hungry. But by employing simple actions such as daily sun exposure, you can activate hunger hormones that suppress the desire to eat more food and powerfully reduce your appetite.

Step 4: Refresh. Even a single night of tossing and turning alters the levels of key satiety and hunger hormones, making you want to eat more than you should. Poor sleep quality also changes how certain motivation centers in your brain react to the sight of food, or even thinking about it. Result: more hunger, more cravings. A good night's sleep—at least two nights a week—is absolutely essential to stop being so effing hungry. When we clean up our sleep habits, we eat normally—and look and feel better.

Step 5: Retrain. To conquer cravings, in particular, you've also got to exercise. Exercising isn't just about training your muscles; it can also regulate neurotransmitters such as dopamine, serotonin, and GABA (gamma-aminobutyric acid) that are intimately involved in our hunger response. If someone suffers from a food addiction, they'll want to pursue dopamine-boosting exercises like outdoor running or yoga. Others might suffer from low serotonin or low GABA. Nature-based exercises are best for those with a serotonin deficiency, while regularly scheduled, set routines are essential for anyone low in GABA. Exercise is a hunger tamer on its own, too, because it reins in the production of hunger hormones. This step is a prescriptive strategy for regulating brain chemicals that affect hunger and cravings.

Breathe a sigh of relief, please! It's absolutely reassuring to know that hunger and cravings are not your fault. And it's even better to know that you can set in motion some easy techniques that don't take much effort but will stop drastic swings in hunger and cravings (and trash eating!), and make you feel satisfied by real food.

In light of everything I've previewed here, treat this book as a critical resource, constant companion, and lifetime guide to a re-freshed and revitalized mind and body. These steps will give you a sense of control and empowerment that ultimately will improve your health, mood, and longevity—and help you appreciate the wonderful body you have.

If you're ready to stop being so effing hungry and start being happy and at peace with your body, let's get started.

# Part I

# The Hunger Puzzle

# 1

# How Did My Hunger Get So Effed Up?

I WAS BORN IN A PART of India called Gujarat, which is described as the Jewel of Western India. It boasts the longest coastline in India and was the home of Mahatma Gandhi, an internationally famous leader known for his nonviolent resistance against British rule.

In Gujarat, the diet is vegetarian, with dishes that are a unique combination of sweet, salty, and spicy (all the flavors we tend to crave!). Fifty years ago, the diet culture in this region was pure, natural, and featured an abundance of unrefined foods. But today, across the board, people are eating fewer fruits, vegetables, and grains—to the detriment of their health—and replacing them with more fat, added sugar, snacks, beverages, and other processed foods introduced to the country by huge food conglomerates like we have in the U.S. They have adulterated the beautiful, traditional diet of my homeland.

Typically, people in Gujarat eat multiple times during the day, starting with a high-carbohydrate breakfast accompanied by tea. Later there's a carb-heavy snack. Lunch is a big meal of rotis and rice, followed by an afternoon snack with more tea. And dinner? You guessed it—a meal heavily loaded with carbs—rice, beans or lentils, and wheat. Yes, there are desserts too, which have a high concentration of sugar.

I remember taking a trip with my uncle and my cousin across Gujarat one summer. They stopped almost every hour or two at different specialty food shops that served up nothing but foods that were fried, refined, and/or full of sugar! At this time, I was a student majoring in nutrition, so it was clear to me that my relatives had developed a sugar addiction. Based on what I had already learned about the neurochemistry of sugar, I also knew it was not their fault. This was sad to me, because people from this region of India commonly develop diseases like diabetes and high cholesterol.

Back home in the U.S., my dad and his brother were struggling with similar issues. They kept a stash drawer filled with candy bars and Indian sweets. They would eat these things to manage their blood sugar when it crashed, instead of taking glucose tablets. But it was more than that. Both had a major sweet tooth and developed intense cravings for sugary food. (By the way, low blood sugar can be better managed by certain combinations of real food—as my dad would later learn.)

Maybe you grew up in a family where rich, carb-laden food was the norm like I did—or your mom made the best desserts in the world. Maybe what you were raised on was a far cry from the healthy, whole, and natural foods of your great-grandparents. Certainly, our food preferences arise from these traditions, as well as from cultural factors. Unlike in the United States, where chocolate is the most craved food, in Japan women are more likely to crave sushi and rice, while in Mexico they often crave tacos. But the influence of cultural and family traditions doesn't tell the whole story of why people get excessively hungry and desire certain foods. It is just a tiny piece of the hunger puzzle.

There's a much bigger piece: a huge web of sneaky signals pulsing throughout your brain, gut, and body that are causing all sorts of havoc on your hunger signals. They largely account for why you get so effing hungry—and why it's not your fault.

# MEET YOUR HUNGER NEURONS

Neurons are cells in your brain and nervous system that relay information to other nerve cells, muscle cells, and gland cells. You are probably thinking: What the eff do nerve cells have to do with me feeling hungry so much? Answer: A lot!

There's a region at the base of your brain called the hypothalamus that has a huge influence on eating behavior. It does other things too. It regulates thirst, various hormones, body temperature, heart rate, and blood pressure, to name a few. One of the master glands of the body (the pituitary is the other), the hypothalamus is the command center that communicates with the rest of the body.

Neuroscientists have zeroed in on a small area of the hypothalamus known as the arcuate nucleus. It is a bundle of fascinating neurons that regulate hunger and satiety: agouti-related protein (AgRP) neurons and proopiomelanocortin (POMC) neurons. (For an informative and fascinating discussion of these neurons and other cellular forces involved in hunger, please listen to the *How Our Hormones Control Our Hunger, Eating & Satiety* podcast by Dr. Andrew Huberman, professor of neurobiology and ophthalmology at Stanford University School of Medicine, at hubermanlab.com.)

These two groups of cells, which collectively occupy an area about the size of a pinhead, are functionally arranged like a seesaw: when AgRP neurons are active, POMC neurons are not, and vice versa. They teeter by releasing chemicals and molecules into the blood that act as accelerators or brakes on the desire to eat and appetite.

When AgRP neurons are doing their thing, we get hungry. As they're firing, they're basically telling you, "You'd better go get food; you're starving."

Imagine you're sitting in your favorite restaurant, hungry and looking forward to your order arriving at your table. The server emerges from the kitchen with a tray full of steaming, delicious food. Anticipation floods over you. But oh no—the server carries the food right past you to another table. Your hunger then really starts raging—at least until you take the first bite of your very own meal.

What's happening is that your AgRP neurons perked up by the sight and even the aroma of the food as it passed by you. When these neurons get stimulated, it's game on. In seconds, your hunger goes through the roof.

The opposing group of neurons, POMC, promotes satiety. When they're active, you feel pleasantly full. Interestingly, lab mice engineered without POMC neurons overeat like crazy and get massively obese because they never receive fullness signals. Similarly, when AgRP neurons are removed from mouse brains, the animals become anorexic and starve themselves.

More specifically, as you get full, POMC neurons suppress your desire to eat by releasing α-melanocyte-stimulating hormone (alpha-MSH) from the pituitary gland. Not well known, alpha-MSH powerfully reduces appetite and is assisted in doing so by leptin, a hunger hormone released from cells in fat tissue.

Alpha-MSH rocks—so naturally we want it to be in balance, and we can do that through some simple behaviors (see the following sidebar "Hunger Hack: Feel Full with More Sunlight").

Another neural mechanism for the brain's hunger and satiety cues involves the vagus nerve. Running from the brain to the gut (intestines, colon, and all the microorganisms within these structures), it is the longest nerve in the human body. It is like a communication superhighway of connectivity between your gut and brain, otherwise known as the gut–brain axis, that sends hunger and satiety messages back and forth. Roughly 90 percent of this communication goes from the gut to the brain and 10 percent from the brain to the gut.

When your stomach gets full, stretch receptors within the stomach communicate with the brain via the vagus nerve to signal satiety. When your stomach is empty, those receptors are inactive.

Based on this information, the brain decides whether you continue or stop eating. According to research in such publications as the *Journal of Neuroendocrinology*, studies have found if the vagus nerve is damaged, one of the outcomes can be obesity, because in the absence of fullness signals emanating from this nerve, people overeat.

The vagus nerve is also involved in cravings for sugar and junk food. There are neurons in your gut that sense sugar intake, and combinations of sugar and fat (like those found in junk food) send subconscious messages to your brain via the vagus nerve. This transmission triggers the release of dopamine, a brain chemical that increases the desire for even more sugar and junk food. In fact, that desire can be so strong that you'll go out of your way to get junk food, like driving to a fast-food restaurant at midnight to get a food fix.

## Hunger Hacks: Feel Full with More Sunlight

The benefits of regular exposure to sunlight are amazing. Sunlight enhances your mood, helps your body make health-protective vitamin D, treats seasonal depression, eases stress, and helps you sleep better at bedtime, among other perks.

I'm adding another benefit to this list: hunger control and satiety!

The reason is that ultraviolet light from the sun activates alpha-MSH—not light absorbed through the skin, but through the eyes. This amazing phenomenon explains why we tend to eat less during spring and summer, but consume more food in the winter months.

For most of us, exposure to sunlight is best first thing in the morning, ideally within the first hour after you crawl out of bed. Spend around a half hour exposing your eyes to sunlight. Don't look directly at the sun, however; this is unsafe. Just being out in the morning sunlight without wearing a sun visor or sunglasses gives you the gentle exposure you need. Going outdoors is key: sunlight through a glass window is far less effective for circadian alignment. So take a morning walk or jog, or sit on your patio or deck while eating breakfast. Don't worry if it's a cloudy day. Even when filtered through clouds, sunlight still offers its hunger-suppressing benefit.

## Hunger, Cravings, and Appetite: What's the Difference?

Is it a craving, or are you just plain hungry? What does it mean to have a big appetite? There are subtle differences among the three, and they involve different pathways in the body.

By definition, hunger is a biological function of the body's real need for food. When you are physically hungry, your stomach, brain, or both prompt you to eat with certain cues. Your stomach may growl, feel empty and hollow, or cause hunger pangs. Your brain may send signals such as a headache, lack of focus, irritability, or brain fog. Some people get physically fatigued or shaky when hungry. Hunger usually doesn't go away over time—it intensifies. There is also a cyclical pattern to hunger cues, depending on the time of day. These are ordinarily a reminder to eat and nourish your body. Only food will satisfy hunger and take the hunger signals away.

Meanwhile, cravings are a powerful desire for food, usually for a specific type of food or drink, such as chocolate, something crunchy or salty, or a dish your mom used to make. Unlike hunger, cravings are not an indication of your body's need for energy. Nor do they elicit hunger cues or result in physical weakness or discomfort if not satisfied.

Cravings can be brought on by hormones, neurotransmitters like dopamine or serotonin, emotions, associations, and memories. Pregnant women also experience cravings for certain types of food; these cravings are often attributed to nutrients that are required during pregnancy.

Aromas can incite cravings. You smell freshly baked doughnuts as you walk past a doughnut shop on the way to work. For a few minutes, you're drawn to their irresistible aroma and you start craving doughnuts.

Appetite is not the same thing as hunger or cravings. Rather, it refers to an interest or disinterest in food and can override hunger and fullness signals. When some people feel stressed or upset over something, they might lose their appetite and choose to ignore signs of hunger.

Others respond the opposite way. Their appetite increases under stress or negative emotions, even if they're not truly hungry. When undergoing a stressful event, have you ever sat down to a delicious meal and continued eating despite feeling full? That, too, is an example of your appetite overriding the signals from your body.

## BRAIN CHEMICALS AND HUNGER

Your hypothalamus not only receives input from hunger neurons, it gets feedback from brain chemicals called neurotransmitters. They carry messages between neurons and other cells in your body, influencing everything from mood to involuntary movements.

There are more than a hundred neurotransmitters in the body, but the two most related to hunger and appetite are serotonin and dopamine. These two neurotransmitters have opposite effects. Low dopamine levels boost hunger, while high serotonin levels suppress it. Therefore, maintaining a balance of both neurotransmitters is important for receiving normal hunger cues and recognizing when you're full.

Dopamine is typically referred to as the reward hormone. It's derived from tyrosine (an amino acid in protein and other foods) and is released when you do competitive things like playing sports or even exercising, as well as having sex or eating a favorite meal.

Too much dopamine, however, causes addictive behaviors because it is a key part of the "reward circuit" in the brain. When a certain behavior like gambling, drinking alcohol, or taking recreational drugs pumps out a lot of dopamine, you feel a pleasurable "high" that you want to reexperience, and so you repeat the behavior. But if you keep repeating that behavior, your brain adjusts to release less dopamine.

The only way to get the same high as before is to engage in even more of the behavior, more often. This is known as substance misuse and leads to addiction.

Eating sugar, which has been integrated into nearly every processed food, releases natural opioids (also called endorphins) and dopamine in our bodies. When you consistently eat foods high in sugar, you can literally get addicted to sugar.

In a study from Connecticut College, researchers showed that Oreo cookies activated the reward circuit in the brains of rats more than cocaine does (and just like humans, the rats ate the filling first). This led to stories in the press about Oreos being more addictive than cocaine. While there were a lot of rats running around high on Oreos, the study results may have been a bit overstated. But we should not take lightly the power of sugar to lure us in, over and over. Sugar most certainly activates opioid receptors and triggers the release of dopamine, and this is one of the reasons food becomes addictive, especially sugar, and is largely responsible for food cravings.

## Cravings Crusher: How to Positively Influence Dopamine

There are ways you can naturally balance dopamine in your body to help control cravings and curb your appetite.

- Eat foods high in tyrosine, such as bananas, almonds, beets, apples, cherries, eggs, meat, and fish. (Oh, and while I'm on the topic of animal proteins, if you eat these foods, make sure they are not processed meats like bologna, salami, hot dogs, deli selections, luncheon meats, among others. These foods are loaded with antibiotics, preservatives, and pesticides that have been linked to inflammation, cardiovascular disease, cancer, high blood pressure, and a whole host of other diseases. Stick to organically raised, hormone-free, antibiotic proteins and grass-fed meats as much as possible.)

- Limit your intake of sugar because it disrupts normal dopamine levels and alters your brain chemistry.
- Do dopamine-balancing workouts such as outdoor cardio or yoga. These are also positive ways to counter food addictions. (I share more on exercise's effect on hormones and neurotransmitters in Chapter 9.)
- Relax and avoid stress. Have a hot bath now and then, get a massage, and meditate to balance your dopamine levels. You may also want to consider starting a stress management program. I offer more information about stress management on my website, at amymdwellness .com/stress.

Serotonin (also known as the happiness hormone) often gets the most attention. It's derived from tryptophan (another amino acid). Much of the serotonin in your body is produced in your gut by the bacteria that reside there. This neurotransmitter provides a sense of happiness and overall well-being. If you find yourself feeling depressed, experiencing insomnia, or low self-esteem, odds are you may need a serotonin boost. Serotonin is the body's natural appetite suppressant. It tames cravings and normalizes your appetite. It makes you feel full even if your stomach is not full, and so you naturally eat less. Having high levels of serotonin can curtail your food intake, but how this happens is not exactly understood. One theory is that serotonin reduces the release of AgRP neurons, which are natural appetite stimulants, and increases the release of alpha-MSH, which suppresses appetite.

**Cravings Crusher:** How to Boost Serotonin Naturally

Serotonin is not only great for your mood and general well-being, it is also helpful for regulating your appetite. It's possible for us to naturally boost our levels of serotonin. Here are some suggestions:

- Eat foods high in tryptophan, including eggs, turkey, dairy foods, lean meats, salmon, pineapples, tofu, nuts, and seeds—but mix them with quality carbohydrates such as sweet potatoes, winter squashes, and quinoa. In fact, I advise that if you add meat or other animal proteins to your diet, they should account for only about 10 percent of the food on your plate.
- Carbohydrates are important because they help drive tryptophan across the blood–brain barrier (BBB), a protective membrane that covers the brain. The BBB prevents toxins from reaching the brain, while allowing vital nutrients to enter.
- Enjoy foods high in vitamin B6, which is important for serotonin production. Plentiful in cauliflower, bananas, avocado, grains, seeds, and nuts, this vitamin must be present to convert tryptophan into serotonin.
- Exercise. When you work out, your body releases more serotonin.
- Get enough sleep, because if you don't, the optimal neurotransmission of serotonin in your system will be disrupted.
- Enjoy sunlight, which will provide you with enough vitamin D to support the synthesis of serotonin.

## THE POWER OF CCK

Hunger is regulated by hormones too. The first hunger hormone to be discovered was cholecystokinin. That's a mouthful, so let's use CCK for shorthand. When released in normal levels by your gut, CCK has a powerful effect on suppressing your appetite. It rises quickly after eating, especially in response to fatty acids, and protein (amino acids).

It's not just any kind of fat that boosts CCK, either. It is a type collectively known as a polyunsaturated fat (PUFA). Polyunsaturated fats are a classification of healthy fats that includes omega-3 and omega-6 fatty acids. Chemically, a PUFA has two or more double bonds in the fatty acid chain while a monounsaturated fat (MUFA) has one double bond.

The journal *Appetite* reported that subjects who followed a diet high in PUFAs for five days had greater levels of CCK than subjects on a high-MUFA diet. In fact, the researchers concluded that "MUFAs did not change any measures of appetite."

If you eat fish, which is packed with omega-3 fatty acids, you will naturally stimulate your body to release CCK, thus blunting your appetite and keeping it at a healthy level. Another type of PUFA that has the same effect is conjugated linoleic acid (CLA), found naturally in meat and dairy and available as a dietary supplement.

A simple, actionable strategy you can take to regulate your hunger and appetite is to include more PUFAs in your diet. The best of the best of PUFAs, in my opinion, are the omega-3s. Great sources are fish and fish oil (mackerel, salmon, sardines, herring, and anchovies), cod liver oil, flaxseed and flax oil, chia, hemp, shrimp, oysters, caviar, and some vegetables (cauliflower, Brussels sprouts).

Another superior source of PUFAs is algae oil, derived from marine algae, and which I prefer because it is vegan. A study in the *Journal of the American Dietetic Association* found algae oil is nutritionally equivalent to cooked salmon and works the same way as fish oil in your body.

Including protein in our meals provides us with amino acids. They can supply energy or be used to build new tissue and repair damaged tissue. They also work to synthesize the hormones we need for communication throughout the body, and they are the building blocks of many of our important neurotransmitters.

If we consume amino acids at the proper levels, along with PUFAs, we can naturally blunt our appetite. Unbeknownst to us, the gut informs the brain via CCK and other mechanisms when we've ingested enough of what we need—PUFAs and amino acids—and tells us we're no longer hungry.

There is one amino acid in particular that directly triggers the release of CCK: glutamine. This amino acid is a critical part of the immune system, where it supplies fuel for infection-fighting white blood cells. It is also an energy source for intestinal cells. Glutamine is found in cottage cheese, eggs, beef, milk, tofu, rice, and corn. Virtually all protein sources contain some glutamine.

Once a threshold of glutamine and other amino acids, plus PUFAs, is reached, CCK is released. It then curtails the activity of the AgRP neurons (discussed earlier) that drive hunger.

As you can see, hunger and appetite control is a well-choreographed dance between your brain, your gut, and your body.

## CCK Public Enemy No. 1: Emulsifiers

When you do your laundry, you dump some detergent into your washing machine along with your dirty clothes. The detergent usually contains emulsifiers to help get rid of stains. By causing a chemical reaction, emulsifiers coat the stain and work to lift it off the fabric.

Food manufacturers put emulsifiers in food, too, particularly prepackaged and processed foods, to make them smoother, creamier, and shelf stable. Think about the last time you made a homemade oil and vinegar salad dressing. It probably began to separate before you put it on the table. Compare that to a store-bought creamy Italian dressing that stays perfectly blended for months. The difference is that emulsifiers in the store-bought dressing prevent its ingredients from separating.

But here's the big problem: When those emulsifiers reach your gut, they strip away its mucosal lining, causing the neurons that innervate the intestines to retreat farther into the gut. Although you are ingesting food, the CCK signals that occur when your body recognizes you are eating and shut down your feeling of hunger never get deployed. Consequently, you want to eat far more of these processed foods than you should because you don't start to feel full. Plus, when emulsifiers adhere to the protective layer of your gut, they cause damage that creates ongoing, low-grade inflammation and changes the protective bacteria in the gut that help manage weight and blood sugar.

All of this creates what we call increased intestinal permeability (aka in lay media as leaky gut), a condition that influences not only digestion but our overall health. With this increased gut permeability, your intestines start to become looser and more porous than usual, and they let food particles seep into your bloodstream. Because your immune system constantly guards the intestinal wall, it sees these particles as intruders and attacks them. Among the many problems with this increased intestinal permeability is that this condition triggers food sensitivities, intolerances, and allergies.

One important remedy to repair the gut is to avoid food processed with emulsifiers—store-bought convenience foods such as mayonnaise, margarine, salad dressings, nut butters, canned frostings, cookies, crackers, creamy sauces, breads, and baked goods. Look around your pantry and read ingredient labels to avoid eating food that contain emulsifiers. Some of the most common are:

Ammonium salt of phosphorylated glyceride
Calcium carbonate
Carboxymethylcellulose
Carrageenan
Casein
Cellulose gum
CSL (calcium stearoyl lactylate)
Glycerol monolaurate
Guar gum
Gum arabic
Lecithin (from soy, sunflower, and egg)
Locust bean gum
Methylcellulose
Mono- and diglycerides
PEG (polyethylene glycol)
PG ester (PGME)
Polyglycerols
Polysorbate 80
PPG (polypropylene glycol)

Sodium potassium tartrate

Sodium stearoyl lactylate

Sorbitan ester (SOE)

Whey protein

Xanthan gum

Above all, minimize the amount of processed foods in your diet. It is virtually impossible to cut out all emulsifiers, because they have infiltrated our foods—even supplements and medications. I eat emulsifiers, but I try to limit them just as I limit processed foods.

Overall, populate your diet with whole, unprocessed foods as much as possible. They are healing to your gut. They help the gut make adhesive proteins that seal the gaps in the intestinal lining, keeping harmful microbes out of the bloodstream, and promoting anti-inflammatory molecules that calibrate your immune system.

I eat a lot of fermented foods as part of my dietary regimen, too—kimchi, sauerkraut, yogurt, kefir, and others, because they help promote gut health (more on this in Chapter 3). The meal plans and nutritional guidelines in this book will help you with all of these nutritional recommendations.

## OTHER KEY HUNGER HORMONES

There are several other hormones intimately connected to hunger besides CCK, most notably leptin and ghrelin. They work together in tandem to suppress or stimulate your hunger and satiety in order to maintain your weight and energy.

Leptin is primarily known as the satiety hormone; its main objective is to keep your body at a healthy weight, and it lets you know that you've had enough food after a satisfying meal.

If you have low levels of leptin, you might feel hungry all the time. This happens with a condition called leptin resistance. Here are a few questions you can use to tell if you may have leptin resistance:

1. Do you have a hard time losing weight?
2. Do you tend to put on weight in your midsection?
3. Are you constantly hungry?
4. Do you frequently crave sugary foods?
5. Are you under a lot of stress?
6. Has your doctor told you that you have high triglycerides and high blood pressure?

So what can you do about leptin resistance? To ensure the best chance at reversing this condition, you must change your diet. Get rid of all processed foods and eat only whole, natural foods, for starters.

---

### Hunger Hack: Balance Leptin

You don't have to be at the mercy of unbalanced leptin. To regulate normal production and prevent a feeding frenzy:

- Log in enough z's. Your body produces leptin while you're sleeping.
- Eat fatty fish a couple of times a week. Good sources are salmon and sardines, which are rich in omega-3 fatty acids, known to increase leptin levels.
- If you are a vegan or vegetarian, supplement your diet with algae oil. Try to choose one that provides at least 250 milligrams of combined EPA and DHA per dosage. Although you can take it at any time of day, I recommend supplementing with a meal—especially one that contains fat, because this macronutrient aids absorption.
- Avoid sugar. Foods high in sugar hinder leptin—and that, my friends, is why you want to eat a whole bag of M&Ms or a box of doughnuts.
- Ease off saturated fats, which cause your body to secrete less leptin. Cut back on high-fat red meats, full-fat cheeses, and other whole-milk products.
- Ease up on your alcohol intake. More than one alcoholic beverage a day for women and more than two for men

---

can make leptin levels drop. Not to mention that a higher alcohol intake can diminish the part of the brain responsible for self-control. With lowered inhibition, you may start to consume more food when drinking alcohol compared to when you're not drinking it.

One more point about alcohol and hunger: you may find that after a night of heavy drinking, the next day you crave something carb- and fat-heavy—say a bacon double cheeseburger. This is a signal that your hunger hormones are out of whack.

Produced in specialized cells located in the lining of your stomach and in the pancreas, ghrelin sends hunger cues to the brain when your stomach is empty, prompting you to eat and store fat to later be turned into energy. It also stimulates the AgRP neurons, making you want to eat.

Ghrelin triggers the reward center in the brain, too, which is why ghrelin is produced when we smell, taste, or even think about tasty foods. Think about the great aromas that waft through the house when your grandmother is cooking Thanksgiving dinner. Your body will start secreting ghrelin in response, and you can't wait to sink your teeth into turkey, stuffing, and mashed potatoes. (You may feel hungry just reading this; that's ghrelin in action too.)

Switching gears a bit, have you ever noticed that you feel hungry at certain times of the day, almost every day? This is the cyclical nature of hunger cues I described earlier. Chalk this up to ghrelin, too. It gets released at the time of day that corresponds with your regular mealtimes. Your stomach will start predictably growling around the normal time of your lunch break or dinner. Even if you've eaten a late breakfast, your system is still accustomed to its normal lunch and dinner slots, and it will release certain ghrelin in anticipation of those habitual times. In short, ghrelin conforms to habitual patterns you've set.

Even though various hormones regulate hunger, you still have the ultimate say in the matter!

## Hunger Hack: Avoid Ultra-Processed Foods to Control Hunger Hormones

In a study published in *Cell Metabolism*, subjects who followed a diet of ultra-processed foods ate about 500 more calories a day and gained weight, compared to when they ate a whole foods diet. Ultra-processed foods included items such as breakfast cereals, muffins, white bread, sugary yogurts, low-fat potato chips, canned foods, processed meats, fruit juices, and diet beverages.

Whole foods are those that remain close to the state you find them in in nature. Examples include fruits, vegetables, legumes, nuts, seeds, and whole grains. Animal foods without additives or processing also fall into this category.

The subjects were recruited by scientists at the National Institutes of Health and fed the ultra-processed diet for two weeks, followed by the whole foods diet for the next two weeks. The researchers prepared all the meals and snacks, tracked their food intake, and carefully analyzed the effects of those foods on the subjects' weight, body fat, and hormones.

Both diets contained roughly equivalent amounts of calories, carbs, fat, and sugar. The subjects were allowed to eat as much as they wanted, and they ended up consuming more calories from the meals when they were given the processed food diet. While on the ultra-processed diet, the subjects gained an average of two pounds of weight gain in two weeks. Almost all of those extra calories came from carbs and fat. On the unprocessed diet, they consumed far fewer calories and lost weight.

What was responsible for these results? Answer: hormones. On the unprocessed diet, their levels of the appetite-suppressing hormone PYY increased while levels of ghrelin, a hormone that stimulates hunger, fell.

So if you want to naturally control your hunger hormones, ease back on processed foods and plan your diet around natural, fiber- and nutrient-rich foods.

## Hunger Hack: Eat Slowly, Feel Full Faster

You've probably heard the advice to eat slowly during a meal in order to feel full, instead of wolfing down your food. Well, this advice holds true, as a result of the many physiological factors that I've talked about in this chapter working in concert.

After you eat or drink a beverage, stretch receptors are activated through the vagus nerve and you start feeling full. As your partially digested meal enters your small intestine from your stomach, hormonal alerts, like those from CCK, sound off in response to the food you ate. Leptin gets into the act, amplifying CCK signals, and tells your brain that you're full. Leptin also interacts with dopamine to enhance feelings of pleasure after eating.

Thus, by eating too fast, you don't give this intricate, well-coordinated hormonal cross talk enough time to do its thing. So slow down at meals, and allow yourself enough time to experience pleasure and satiety.

## THE INSULIN, GLUCOSE, AND GLUCAGON CONNECTION

Because so many members of my family have been diagnosed with type 2 diabetes, I have a lot of personal experience with the hormone insulin. In this form of diabetes, there is a gradual breakdown in the mechanisms that handle glucose in the body. Glucose accumulates to toxic levels in the blood, and the pancreas can't make enough insulin to keep up. So there isn't sufficient insulin to do the job of helping cells take up glucose for fuel. That's type 2 diabetes in a nutshell.

But under normal, healthy conditions, insulin helps cells function by feeding them blood sugar for energy. Let's say you eat a potato. The carbohydrates in that potato are broken down into glucose and passed into the bloodstream. The pancreas detects the release of glucose and will start to secrete insulin into the bloodstream to collect the glucose and deliver it to your cells for energy.

Too much insulin can create a condition known as insulin resistance. How does this happen exactly? When you eat a sugary meal, your insulin levels shoot up, and if you constantly eat sugary meals, day after day, your pancreas will continue to produce too much insulin. Picture this scenario as a mother (insulin) who yells at her small child (our cells) morning and night. After a while, the child starts to ignore the yelling, and the cellular receptors don't take in the insulin they should—they resist.

Insulin resistance causes lots of worrisome health issues, including cardiovascular disease, type 2 diabetes, and Alzheimer's disease. For the purposes of our discussion around hunger, know that with insulin resistance, you'll experience increased hunger, crave sugary foods, and eat more than you should.

The pancreas's second main hormone, glucagon, helps insulin by working as an opposing force. When you're hungry, you secrete glucagon. It prompts your cells to release glucose from your liver and muscles. After those stores are depleted, glucagon will unlock body fat for energy. Glucagon is also a weight-loss hormone.

---

## Hunger Hack: Stop Overeating with One Simple Trick

Naturally, you want this push-pull system of insulin and glucagon to work as it should in order to keep your hunger levels in check. The good news is that this is pretty easy to do, as long as you eat your protein, carbohydrates, and fat (the macronutrients) in a specific order at meals.

Let me give you an example. How often have you been seated at a restaurant and the waitperson sets before you a basket of rolls or a loaf of bread? Pretty standard practice, right? Well,

---

eating a carb right before a meal stimulates a big release of glucose, and with it, a surge in dopamine. The net effect is to make you want to consume even more food at the meal.

Alcohol, by the way, triggers the same physiological reactions because it is high in sugar. I know, I know, you don't want me to say this, but sipping a few cocktails while nibbling on bread in the restaurant before eating your main meal will mess up your hunger signals big time!

If you want to achieve satiety earlier in your meal, eat your food in this order:

1. A fibrous vegetable like a salad or green veggie.
2. The protein and healthy fat portion of your meal.
3. The carbohydrate, such as a potato or a serving of rice.

By preventing steep rises in your glucose, the order in which you eat your food has enormous impact on hunger and fullness.

The evidence is overwhelming that cravings and an out-of-control appetite and hunger are not your fault. But there's so much more to these issues than the physiological factors I've just discussed—a whole lot more. For now, start practicing my hunger hacks and cravings crushers, and you'll begin to free yourself from the grip of these issues. In the next chapter, we'll look at how emotions and societal influences shoulder the blame too—and make us sometimes feel like no matter how much we eat, we can never get enough.

# 2

## The Hunger Hijackers

I WILL NEVER FORGET THE FIRST conversation I had with Katie, a dentist, part owner of her practice, and a mom to four young children. Week by week, she struggled with hunger and cravings, while trying to shed pounds. She was always trying to follow a restrictive, low-carb diet. From Monday to Wednesday, she stuck to that plan. But by the time Thursday rolled around, Katie was pooped, she couldn't sleep, and she craved salty foods like chips and crackers. She shared with me that one Friday night, to unwind, she went to a Mexican restaurant with friends. She had a large margarita, plus devoured almost the whole basket of tortilla chips put on the table before the meal. But she also confessed that this wasn't the first time for the indulgence; this eating behavior had become a pattern in her life.

But it didn't stop there. Each Saturday morning, she would wake up feeling so ashamed that she would drive to the grocery store and purchase a bag of chips and eat them in frustration. Then, come Sunday, Katie started slashing carbs again on her low-carb diet.

Meanwhile, she hoped and prayed that her family would not notice this cycle of dieting then overeating. She asked me during our appointment, "Why can't I control this? I'm tired of feeling guilty and inadequate. I'm tired of this vicious cycle that I know is really destructive."

When the going got tough, Katie—like countless other women I've treated—was known to get eating. Can you relate? A tight deadline at work? Grab that bag of chips. The mortgage overdue? Where are the fudge brownies? Your teen constantly breaking curfew? Pass that third glass of wine, please.

Katie is the perfect victim of what I call a hunger hijacker. There are three big ones.

The first is emotional eating, driven by feelings of stress, anxiety, anger, depression, loneliness, or even joy. The second is the modern food environment. Food manufacturers have purposely engineered foods to be ultrapalatable, even addictive substances that make us want to eat more, especially when we're stressed out or feeling other intense emotions. Third is the diet industry, which has created guilt and other negative feelings about food and our bodies and produced the opposite intended effect—weight gain, obesity, and poor health.

These hunger hijackers are also intertwined with the physiological factors I talked about in the previous chapter; they deeply affect the brain, messing with hunger signals. Like those physiological factors, hunger hijackers are another reason why you're so effing hungry and why none of this is your fault.

## FOOD AND EMOTIONS

When you eat to make yourself feel better and avoid feeling difficult emotions, this is called emotional eating. If you're an emotional eater, you've probably stressed yourself out more by thinking, like Katie did, that you must fix your emotional eating problem. Well, the good news is that this so-called problem is not your fault either. I repeat: emotional eating is not your fault. Read on to understand why.

## Early Conditioning

Many of us have been conditioned from infancy to respond to discomfort or feelings of pain through food. When babies cry, they get sweet, fatty milk, and they are happy again. When we fall and scrape our knees, our moms give us ice cream or a lollipop to comfort us. When we go to Grandma's house, she makes our favorite foods for us.

From an early age, we have learned that when we are feeling down or sad, food can make us feel better. As adults, we want to go back to that feeling of being cradled in our mother's arms, feeling loved, safe, and secure. So we reach for foods that mimic that early biochemical desire to bond with Mom and other early childhood experiences.

As we get older, our brains become cross-wired as a result of this early conditioning, and we eat in response to any discomfort that comes along. Food becomes the soother of emotional pain.

## Trauma

Some people engage in unhealthy eating behaviors to push away painful emotions and stress caused by trauma—an accident, sexual or emotional abuse, domestic violence, personal loss or tragedy, a pandemic, or a wartime experience. Traumatic experiences actually rewire the brain, sometimes causing us to feel excessively stressed, even when there's nothing apparent to stress over. What's more, studies show that trauma can shrink the hippocampus—the brain region that controls appetite and regulates emotions.

When trauma keeps hitting us, cortisol—the hormone secreted during times of stress—can flood the brain. Cortisol activates a region in the brain called the amygdala. It is responsible for emotions and emotional behavior (like overeating). When this happens, even more cortisol can be churned out. That's bad news on several levels, but for our purposes here, know that cortisol influences several hormones involved in hunger and cravings. These include leptin, insulin, and neuropeptide Y (NPY). Cortisol also suppresses the production of serotonin, which helps control hunger, cravings, and appetite. The net effect of all this havoc is that you're more likely to overindulge or eat without thinking.

## The Loneliness Effect

Any intense feeling can bring on emotional eating, but loneliness is really rough on appetite control—and some fascinating research proves this. In the journal *Nature and Neuroscience*, scientists at MIT reported that being alone for ten straight hours caused activity in the brain similar to going without food for ten hours. In other words, people desired social contact just like they desired food when they were hungry. In fact, dopamine neurons in the reward circuit of the brain lit up more when people viewed photographs of both food and friends after they had been deprived of those things.

This research underscores the importance of staying connected with others. If just one day of being alone makes our brains respond as if we had not eaten for a whole day, this suggests that close relationships are a very basic need that we have and it should be fulfilled.

---

### Hunger Hacks: Manage Emotional Eating

You don't have to be at the mercy of emotional eating. You can rein in undesirable eating habits and keep them in check. To help stop emotional eating, I have the following suggestions for you.

*Keep a food diary.* I think it's extremely helpful and eye-opening to keep a journal of your diet. Write down the foods you eat, the quantity, the times you eat them, how you feel when eating these foods, and how hungry you feel. Eventually, you'll begin to see patterns between your mood and food. You can break these patterns by having substitute activities (other

---

than eating) when you feel emotional, such as exercising, reading, or doing a fun hobby.

*Work on your stress levels.* If stress triggers emotional overeating, pursue a stress management technique you like—maybe yoga, meditation, or deep breathing. The latter is one of my favorite ways to manage cortisol levels. Try this exercise: take three long breaths—six counts in and six counts out. You'll feel the stress-relieving difference almost immediately.

*Remove food cues.* These are signals, or prompts, in our environment that get us to eat. The idea that these cues trigger hunger is nothing new. Remember Ivan Pavlov and his dogs? As early as 1905, Pavlov conditioned dogs to salivate (a hunger sign) when they heard a bell. Cues are powerful but not unchangeable. Start by rearranging the environment in which you live and work. Stock your kitchen with nutrient-rich foods, don't keep hard-to-resist foods like sweets or salty snacks around, or change your commute to avoid driving by your favorite burger joint. And if you feel angry or depressed, put off going grocery shopping until you have your emotions in check. These actions reprogram your environment and set you up for success.

*Move your body.* You can soothe a mental funk by getting regular exercise. A walk or jog around your neighborhood or a quickie yoga routine may help in particularly emotional moments.

*Strengthen your social connections.* Get together more often with friends and family when possible. Join social groups in which you share interests or volunteer for causes in which you'll interact with others. Just don't isolate; be around people you care about.

*Learn from slips and relapses.* If you have a setback, don't dwell on it. Forgive yourself and begin anew the next day. Learn from your experience and make a plan for preventing it next time. Focus on the positive changes you're making and congratulate yourself for the successes you've made to date.

# THE MODERN FOOD ENVIRONMENT

The food industry makes more profit from processed food than it does from healthy, unprocessed food. Hence, companies engineer food products in various ways, from ingredients to packaging, that make food emotionally and physically triggering on purpose.

When you go grocery shopping, it's overwhelming to see cravings-promoting, processed, and junk foods galore stocked on the shelves (read more about this below). Interestingly, only a handful of powerful companies produce these foods and they have the market share of 80 percent of grocery items that Americans purchase regularly, according to joint investigation by the *Guardian* and Food and Water Watch. Those companies are Kraft, General Mills, Conagra, Unilever, and Del Monte. Their goal is to dominate the market, or what food industry insiders call grabbing stomach share.

The power wielded by these Big Food companies largely dictates what the 2 million farmers in the U.S. grow and how much they get paid, as well as what people eat and how much our groceries cost. One problem is that they have squeezed out many small-scale farmers, regional food hubs, and grocery co-ops, all of which tend to produce healthier, less processed foods. What's really scary to me is that these companies have bought up many of the natural and organic food companies.

The biggest problem, though, is that these giants create and push foods so intoxicating that we addictively crave their deviously developed products. They add hunger-stimulating substances to foods to make us eat more, they manipulate flavor to get us to wolf down processed and fast foods, and they package and advertise foods in a way that sends consumers the message that certain food products will make us happy, confident, and loved.

The highly processed foods made by these companies also spike glucose levels. If we eat these foods consistently, they then cause our glucose levels to fall after spiking, sending our insulin levels on a roller-coaster ride. In general, we are eating too much junk, and we are not eating enough prebiotic fiber and vegetables.

(We need prebiotics to encourage the growth of good gut bacteria, which have a lot to do with hunger and satiety. More on this in Chapter 3.)

Even worse, highly processed foods trick the mind and hoodwink our hunger signals. Those pancakes at the pancake house or the pizza from your favorite delivery place may be delicious, but they are low in protein, an essential nutrient that keeps our blood sugar levels stable, which in turn helps create that feeling of fullness by reducing levels of ghrelin (the hormone that tells us to eat).

## Food Additives and Alterations

Unbeknownst to a lot of us, the foods we buy have additives lurking in them or they have otherwise been altered in ways that actually make us hungrier and hijack the brain to make our emotional eating worse. The unfortunate thing is that if you are not aware of this problem, and you don't know what to look for, there's a good chance you won't notice what's been added to the foods you eat. However, by knowing about food additives and alterations, and understanding how to read a food label, you can do your body a whole world of good. Here's a look.

- Monosodium glutamate (MSG). Added to 80 percent of flavored foods, MSG antagonizes your pancreas into pouring out more insulin—a hormonal cascade that makes you feel hungry. MSG has also been shown to negatively impact your hypothalamus, which regulates leptin, your I'm-full hormone. It has also been linked to diabetes and obesity and is even considered an excitotoxin. This means that MSG makes brain cells get overexcited, and then they fire uncontrollably, leading to cell death. Although there is definitely controversy surrounding the science, if you find MSG on the label of something you're about to eat, skip it.
- Refined flour. The word "refined" in flour refers to a modification process in which the bran and germ are removed,

allowing products to stay on the shelves longer. However, this process also removes the naturally occurring vitamins, minerals, and dietary fiber.

Refined flour, mainly white flour, jacks up your blood sugar levels fast, spiking your insulin levels and then making them crash. The reaction makes you hungry again very quickly. This is why you may feel like eating again soon after having a bagel or a slice of toast.

• Refined sugar. White sugar works on the body in a very similar way to refined flour. It sends your blood sugar sky-high and then makes it crash a short time later, intensifying your craving for more sugar. Once you start eating it, it can be difficult to stop.

Sugar can also make you briefly feel high (as in "on a drug") and creates a spark of energy in your body because of the dopamine release it brings.

A particularly vile form of refined sugar is high fructose corn syrup. Laced into sodas, commercial juices, and other beverages as well as packaged foods, high fructose corn syrup messes up your normal metabolism. Its chemical structure is engineered to make you keep eating more and more of it. Studies have found that this additive slows down the release of leptin, the I'm-full hormone.

• Gluten. Back to white bread for a moment: Another reason it makes you hungry is its gluten content. Gluten is a protein in wheat that is often present in processed foods. It can be highly inflammatory in certain groups of people because of its sugar-like properties when refined, and it is also a gut irritant.

If you are intolerant to gluten, you may experience hormonal imbalances and nutritional inadequacies that make you feel insatiable and ill at the same time. Gluten also breaks down into opiate-like substances called gluteomorphin and casomorphine, which act on opiate receptors. If you suspect you are addicted to food and eat emotionally, a gluten intolerance might be one of the explanations.

**Cravings Crusher:** Goodbye, Gluten

There is a lot of controversy around whether we should be eliminating gluten across the board. A good rule of thumb is to avoid gluten-containing products for a month. See what happens and how you feel. Note whether you are in better control of hunger, cravings, and emotional eating. Personally, gluten was a hidden food sensitivity for me, and I do better without it. Because of the decreased nutritional value in most grains, they should be a small part of our diets anyway.

## The Science of Flavor

In the processed food industry, employing scientists to tinker with the ratios of salt, sugar, and fat to optimize taste is standard operating procedure. Some critics feel that these practices have hooked people on their products almost as much, say some critics, as the tobacco industry has gotten smokers addicted to nicotine. Much of the food we buy in this country is, in fact, the result of an engineering project.

Science has shown that addiction centers of the brain are activated by high glycemic index foods, which cause your blood sugar to rise quickly. Incorporating enough sugar into a food to activate these areas is a top priority in food engineering projects.

How exactly do food scientists come up with the foods we like and crave the most? I talked about bliss point in the introduction. It refers to a specific recipe of three nutrients: fat, sugar, and salt. In combination, all three stimulate our thousands of tastebuds and tell the brain that we need to eat more and more of this particular food. Many natural, unprocessed foods such as fresh fruit also contain these three nutrients, though not in the ideal bliss point ratio that keeps us coming back for more.

Bliss point also enhances mouth feel so that the taste sensation makes food irresistible. For example, fat imparts a smooth texture for the perfect mouth feel to foods like chips and crackers.

Within the bliss point formula, at least 50 percent of the calories of a food generally come from fat to activate a pleasure response from eating the food. Salt disguises the chemical flavor of junky foods and is the cheapest spice around. Sugar stimulates the reward and pleasure centers in our brains.

Food manufacturers thus tinker with fat, sugar, and salt, and then exhaustively taste test their concoctions until they reach the perfect bliss point and mouth feel so that consumers succumb to their cravings and eat more of that food product. The higher a food's craving level, the more sales and profit it generates.

One fascinating example of this kind of research has to do with Dr Pepper soda. While working to come up with a brand-new product, the company experimented with sixty-one formulas and held four thousand taste tests. Throughout these tests, food scientists constantly tweaked the recipe until they arrived at the perfect bliss point. The result? Cherry Vanilla Dr Pepper, one of the company's most successful products ever.

So you see, food companies are purposefully hijacking our brains with the foods that they create. They want to create a pleasure experience so intense that you continually purchase their products, and, in essence, become addicted to the specific formulation of salt, sugar, and fat in them. They're robbing you of your ability to easily make food choices because you're returning to foods from which you experience pleasure, even when you know better.

By being aware of how the food industry contributes to hunger and cravings, poor health, increased stress, and astronomical health care costs, we can make different choices and be the change in our lives, our families' lives, and the health of our communities.

## Food Advertising

Let me focus here on a couple of highly processed food products that really irk me—packaged snacks and cereals. Snacks haul in huge profits, thanks to more than $10 billion spent yearly by the food industry on snack food advertising. Many of these snacks are hyperpalatable foods that can stimulate reward circuits in the brain. I'm talking about craveable products that include potato chips, crackers, ice cream, soda, and candy, all formulated to tell the brain: "Eat me!"

Then there are advertising shenanigans that go on right in your favorite grocery store. I consider myself a pretty savvy, informed shopper who makes food decisions based on my nutritional training and preferences. So when I learned that grocery stores use specific strategies to influence my spending, I was miffed and intrigued at the same time. This has been researched extensively, with studies concluding that what you see is what you'll buy: you're more likely to take home food that is shelved at eye level. Looking up, looking down, bending over, or reaching for an item requires additional effort and may keep us from purchasing it.

And advertising reaches kids, too—they can get very attracted to cereals that have cartoon characters on their boxes! As a mom to two children, I now think twice about taking my kids down the cereal aisle. Also, wouldn't it be great if manufacturers of healthier breakfast choices could add a cartoon character to the box to make their cereal more appealing to our children?

## Food Containers

Eating and drinking are intense pleasurable experiences that involve the appearance, aroma, texture, and taste of foods and beverages— and the food industry knows this. Another thing they know is that color is very important to how we perceive food, drink, and meals in general. Now, research indicates that the color of containers has a huge and subtle impact on how much we consume.

Open your cupboard and look at the color of your coffee mugs and dinner plates. Why? Because I think you'll find these next pieces of research to be rather eye-opening.

A study published in 2014 in *Flavour* examined the effect of mug color on people's taste for coffee. The participants were served identical coffees in either a white ceramic, blue ceramic, or clear glass mug and asked to rate these characteristics of the coffee in each mug: quality, aroma, bitterness, sweetness, and acceptability.

Those who drank from a white mug described the coffee as more intense and bitter than did those who drank from the clear glass mug, while the coffee in the blue mug was perceived as somewhere in between. The participants thought the coffee served in the clear glass and blue mugs tasted sweeter than coffee consumed from the white mugs.

Interesting, right? So what's the deal?

The researchers theorized that "it's not the whiteness of the cups that matters per se, but rather the way it brings out the clarity and vividness of the brownness of the coffee, which tends to be associated with bitter flavors."

But container color doesn't only impact the perception of taste; it can also affect how much food we eat. In a study published in *Appetite*, participants were served the same amounts of popcorn and chocolate chips on red, blue, or white plates. The researchers then observed that participants ate less popcorn and chocolate when eating off a red plate.

However, if the food was red and the plate was red too, consumptive habits could be different. Published in *The Nutrition Journal*, one study found that test subjects in a buffet line served themselves 22 percent more pasta with marinara sauce when using red plates versus white plates.

So the next time you find yourself lounging on your sofa, drinking from a blue mug or eating red Starburst candy from a red bowl, with your hand in an empty potato chip bag, blame the food industry!

## The Diet Industry

Nearly 45 million of us start a diet every year, and we collectively spend $33 billion annually on weight-loss products, according to the Boston Medical Center and reported in the American Council on Science and Health. Yet, nearly two-thirds of Americans are overweight or obese.

One reason is the diet industry, which profits mostly when people get—and stay—overweight. As I noted in the introduction, there's no money to be made if everyone in society maintains a stable, healthy weight.

The diet industry has hijacked and sabotaged us in a number of ways. It has:

- Taught us to deny and dismiss our hunger cues and rely instead on lists of food to eat, when, and in what portions.
- Told us that hunger is bad. Hunger is an important messenger, and killing the messenger doesn't erase the message that it's time to eat, which we need to do to stay alive.
- Fed us the idea that we can control our hunger with discipline and willpower (NOT!).
- Created guilt and other negative feelings about food and our bodies.

One of the big hunger-related issues with dieting is that most diets pressure us to restrict a lot of foods, calories, and sometimes whole food groups like carbohydrates. If you're not getting enough calories, your brain releases neuropeptide Y (NPY), a hormone that makes you crave carbohydrates. This response is basically your body's innate survival mechanism kicking in to make sure you have all the fuel you need to get stuff done.

Also, if you've been dieting and restricting foods that give you pleasure—say, pizza, cookies, or your favorite ice cream—you're going to not only be more apt to eat those foods, particularly after a stressful day at work, but also more inclined to overeat them.

Studies reveal that the reward circuits in your brain light up even more in response to a food that has been previously off-limits. So that ice cream you buried in the depths of your freezer? You might eat more of it if you restrict it than if you allow yourself some scoops on occasion and in moderation.

Also, the diet industry, through social media, celebrity magazines, and some TV programs, likes to talk about weight and food issues in moral terms, such as: "I've been good today, I didn't eat the muffin at work." But if someone feels guilty and ashamed when they eat something they enjoy and deny themselves all their favorite foods, they will obviously feel bad. What does someone who tends to emotionally eat do when they feel bad? They eat, of course.

The diet industry further bombards us with images and comparisons that promote a negative body image if we don't meet its standards. Advertising is designed to make you believe that you need the diet-industry companies' products to look good. But what you need is self-compassion—being kind and accepting of yourself.

Yes, the food and diet industries have hijacked our taste buds and our brain chemistry, and made it easier to turn to food to soothe our emotions. But in my 5-step program, I will show you the keys to breaking free from cravings and stop being so effing hungry all the time (and subsequently you can use these tools and apply them to other areas of your life).

This is exactly what happened to Katie. It was clear to me that she was a victim of hunger hijackers, and all of her hunger signals were off. I put her on my plan and encouraged her to incorporate as many of my hunger hacks and cravings crushers as she could. After only one month, Katie came back, excited to report her progress. "This has been amazing. I crave salty foods significantly less often, and I have no desire to eat emotionally. I'm in a better mood and less stressed. The healthy foods I now enjoy fill me up naturally, and I feel great."

With Katie, we can see how hidden influences—in the ways the body and brain work and how we're being manipulated by outside forces—reroute all of our hunger-appetite pathways. Just as my plan helped Katie, the good news is that for you, too, those pathways can be normalized to help you naturally and effortlessly get your own hunger and cravings under control.

There is one final piece of the hunger puzzle that I want to tell you about—psychobiotics—that explains a lot about why you can't just eat one of those chips. That's where we're headed next.

# 3

# The Power of Psychobiotics

**D**URING OUR FACETIME CALL, ROBERT described to me his embarrassing yet uncomfortable symptoms. "Right after I eat, I inflate like a balloon," said the 42-year-old tax accountant as he ticked off his complaints. "Then there's this terrible gassy feeling. I'm lucky if this gas results in a belch, but more often than not, it escapes in a different direction, if you know what I mean."

I certainly did. Millions of people struggle regularly with distress after eating, including bloating, gas, abdominal pain, or diarrhea. After food, especially processed carbs, enters the small intestine largely undigested, it moves on to the colon. There, bacteria begin to dismantle the undigested food particles, a process that causes gas due to fermentation.

For doctors, the origin of stomach problems like Robert's can be difficult to determine. They can arise from any number of underlying conditions, and they are becoming increasingly common. Most problems lead to a diagnosis of exclusion, meaning they fall into the vague category of what illnesses are left when other possibilities are ruled out.

But everything Robert was telling me—uncomfortable bloating and gas after a meal—gave me a strong hunch that he was suffering from a buildup of bad gut bacteria—a condition called dysbiosis. Sometimes these symptoms can be normal, but not if you're experiencing them every day like Robert was. His gut was trying to communicate with him and doing a pretty good job.

Despite being normally good humored, Robert was indeed, desperate. In a rare moment of seriousness, he confessed, "I will try anything."

Having had Robert as a patient for some time, I knew that the treatment—which would largely involve dietary changes—would be challenging. Robert had intense sugar cravings and found desserts irresistible, especially in response to the pressures of his high-stress job. Also, his frequent consumption of desserts was one reason that he had a tough time keeping weight off. I explained to him that some bacteria thrive on sugar, and too much sugar can cause an imbalance in the digestive tract and lead to several gut issues.

Study after study reveals that our gut microbes exert a great deal of influence on health conditions ranging from autoimmune disorders to allergies and obesity. And diet is the number-one reason why.

With patients like Robert, I always emphasize the health-damaging effects of a standard Western diet, which is notoriously low in the fiber that nourishes gut microbes. Our bodies have really not evolved to handle this kind of diet. Meals full of processed foods cause the steep rises in blood sugar that can lead to diabetes and other chronic diseases over time. Eating less natural, fiber-rich foods in favor of more refined, high-sugar carbs causes the decline of healthy microbes and the proliferation of bad bacteria that make us sick in many ways.

I worked with Robert to slowly change his diet, strictly monitor it, and wean him off sugar and processed foods. He started adding more vegetables at every meal, eating more fermented foods, and taking in other nutrients known to help curb cravings. All of this helped enormously. He felt better and lost 25 pounds in just three months. "In a way, I'm like a different person now," he told me, looking back on the symptoms that once dominated his life. He is convinced that by simply changing his diet, he had found a cure.

The connection between gut health and overall well-being has been proven again and again—which is why I advise my patients to take it seriously, especially if you have trouble with cravings and are hungry all the time. If you're like Robert and many other people, the struggle to resist foods that are high in sugar, fat, or salt (or all of the above) is a part of your daily life. And it may seem like these eating patterns can be tough to change. It sure doesn't help when we're told that it's a problem of self-control or lack of willpower—of course, this is all nonsense, as I've mentioned earlier.

You already know that there are neurons, brain chemicals, hormones, and other physiological factors involved in hunger, cravings, and appetite. Emotions get in the way too, along with a few other things that make us hungry: aroma, the sight of food, reading or thinking about it, even fond memories of delicious meals. As do cues that seem unrelated to food: the sofa where you always watch TV while munching on buttered popcorn, a social event like a New Year's Eve party, or a trip to your favorite shopping mall.

Add in the fact that the food and diet industries are conspiring against us to trigger our hunger-control systems and drive up our appetites with craveable foods that are relatively cheap and full of sugar, empty calories, and fat.

Before we get to my 5-step plan, let's jump into another reason why hunger and cravings are not your fault: your microbiome—the ecosystem of all microbes, such as bacteria, fungi, viruses, and their genes, that naturally live on our bodies and within us.

One of the important concepts now emerging from the study of microbiome health is referred to as psychobiotics. This term collectively describes living organisms that, when ingested in the right quantities, produce a benefit for mental health, mood, behavior (including eating behavior), and appetite. To better understand psychobiotics in terms of eating behavior, let's first take a look at what goes on inside the gut.

# GUTSY REACTIONS

In the womb, we don't have a single microbe in our developing guts. But as we pass through our mother's birth canal, we begin to build entire colonies of bacteria. By the time we can crawl, our little guts have become even more populated by microbes—a hundred trillion or more. We pick them up from practically everywhere: the food we eat and contact with other people, furniture, clothing, cars, our homes and other buildings, soil, pets, even the air we breathe.

Microbes take up residence in the gut and mouth, all over the skin, and in the lining of the throat. As many as ten thousand bacterial species inhabit our bodies, outnumbering our own cells by ten to one and weighing about three pounds—the same as the brain—and they play a crucial role in our health.

Some are good bacteria; others are bad. This may come as a surprise, because we typically portray bacteria as bad guys that try to make us sick, and we fight them off with antibiotics and antibacterial products like hand sanitizers, wipes, and soaps, all designed to ward off these nasty buggers. Antibiotics have saved countless lives, but it is very important that we not lose sight of the fact that their overuse can annihilate good bacteria as well as bad. Without most of those good guys, we could not survive.

The vast majority of the microbes in the body encamp in our gut, and that's where issues involving hunger, cravings, and appetite arise. This is why getting your gut in healthy working condition can stop you from being so effing hungry all the time.

We've known for a while that the good bacteria are necessary for our health. But what exactly do they do for us?

They work constantly on our behalf. Their main function is to consume certain types of carbohydrates and other nutrients that make their way through the gut. This process produces short-chain fatty acids (acetate, butyrate, and propionate—sometimes called postbiotics) that your body uses for fuel and other important functions.

Microbes patrol our guts to prevent infections; they help to form and strengthen our immune system and digest food. Some recent studies have found that gut bacteria may even modify our brain chemistry, thus affecting our moods and behavior.

These good bacteria also manufacture vitamins, including the energy-supporting B vitamins, like B12, thiamine, and riboflavin; as well as vitamin K2, which is needed for normal blood coagulation. Some bacteria regulate your metabolism, which tells you when you're hungry, full, or need that midafternoon snack.

Other vital compounds are produced by good gut bacteria, too—like serotonin, the feel-good neurotransmitter that is involved in controlling hunger and cravings. As much as 80 to 90 percent of serotonin is synthesized in the microbiome, as well as 50 percent of dopamine. Our gut microbiome also synthesizes hormones, including the sleep-promoting hormone melatonin.

As long as the good bacteria outweigh the bad, you'll enjoy high energy levels, a healthy digestive tract, strong immunity, a clear and focused mind—and normal hunger signals and fewer cravings.

## HUNGER GAMES

Do you have kids involved in sports or are you an athlete yourself? Well, gut microbes are a lot like athletes who participate in team sports. Their lives are structured like a game in which players compete for the various resources that are at stake. With gut microbes, those stakes are nutrients and space. The more diverse the team of microbes, the more successful they are at accessing those resources—like a team of players with the best and broadest range of athletic skills. So basically, an ongoing all-star game is occurring daily in your digestive system as differing species of bacteria compete for available nutrients and territory. This is one of the reasons that a highly diverse microbiome is a healthy one, because it ensures there is no room for pathogenic bacteria to muscle their way in.

That diversity, however, is constantly at risk because our Western culture, diet, and lifestyle have caused a decrease in the wonderful composition of our microbiome. Added sugar, processed food, poor sleep quality, and even chronic stress can all wreck the gut. Recent studies have also demonstrated that there is a connection between the decrease in the microbiome's bacterial content and an increase in obesity. Interestingly, people with obesity often have less microbial diversity than those who maintain a healthy weight. This may partially explain why many people who are overweight struggle with food cravings (poor gut diversity contributes to cravings—see "Hunger Hack: Diversify Your Microbes in One Easy Step" below).

Scientists now speculate that an imbalance of microbes in the gut might be a major barrier to weight loss.

Dwindling bacterial diversity has also led to an increase in auto-immune diseases, gastrointestinal illnesses, and other conditions seen in countries like the U.S., where the diets are high in sugar and fat and low in fiber intake.

By contrast, the more types of bacteria you have, the healthier you are. We thus need a healthy, diverse population of bacteria to keep our bodies functioning optimally. You'll learn how to accomplish this when we get to my 5-step plan.

Bacteria aren't much for individual sports, either. They don't like being lonely and need to know they are not alone. Like humans, they need to talk to each other, socialize, and interact with other bacteria. To do so, they use a mechanism called quorum sensing, which involves special molecules that emit signals to talk to other bacteria. A quorum refers to the number of other bacteria in the surrounding area. So, through quorum sensing, a bacterium knows exactly how many other bacteria are in their neighborhood.

Scientists are learning more about how quorum sensing may be one way in which microbes coordinate their behavior to manipulate our eating habits to enhance their own nutritional supply.

---

## Hunger Hack: Diversify Your Microbes in One Easy Step

One important aspect of psychobiotics is the addition of probiotics—good bacteria—to your diet. These can rein in your

---

food intake, diversify your microbiome, and even help you shed pounds. Probiotics provide a great amount of nutrients and phytochemicals.

Reported in the *American Journal of Clinical Nutrition*, a study of yogurt showed that it had the most impact on weight loss after researchers monitored the diets and health of 120,000 nurses over a span of twelve to twenty years. Yogurt is a fermented food and a good source of probiotics.

A word of caution: A trend in recent years from the food industry is to add probiotics to all kinds of foods, from juices to energy bars. Ultimately, most are not effective and thus are a huge waste of your money. In fact, it can be impossible to know what you're getting when you buy a probiotic-formulated product.

For best results, reap the benefits of probiotics by drinking kombucha, coconut kefir, or other fermented foods, or eating a natural yogurt to which probiotics have not been added. As for yogurt, Greek strains of yogurt are relatively high in natural probiotics (but beware much of the processed yogurt on the market is devoid of probiotics—read the label).

## GUT MICROBES ARE PICKY EATERS

Like you, different microbes like to munch on different kinds of foods. Although many microbes are generalists and can thrive on a variety of nutrients, most typically prefer one kind of food over another.

For example, Bacteroidetes enjoy fats; *Prevotella* love carbs; and *Bifidobacteria* crave dietary fiber. Other gut bugs are really picky and feed only on a single nutrient. Some microbes, such as *Akkermansia muciniphila,* don't rely on food sources at all but prefer the carbohydrate secreted by the mucous layer of your gut lining. This preference is actually a survival mechanism: the human intestine evolved to produce food for beneficial gut bacteria, assuring that they can thrive and survive even during long fasts. Without this strong, defensive barrier of mucus and friendly bacteria, the human body is very susceptible to infectious disease.

Do you have any idea what the disease-promoting bacteria like to eat? You guessed it—sugar! When we eat a diet high in refined, added sugar, undesirable bacteria thrive and start growing out of control, while our beneficial bacteria decline in number and diversity. Because the standard Western diet is so loaded with added sugar, poor gut diversity is a big health risk for many people.

## GOT CRAVINGS? BLAME YOUR GUT!

When you feel overcome by food cravings, the cause can have a lot to do with the bacteria in your gut. A fascinating study from the University of California, San Francisco reviewed dozens of studies on the human microbiome and found that it can dictate the kinds of foods you crave.

But how can these invisible critters drive you to feed on candy or chips or some other food? According to the researchers, they do so by tapping into the nerve pathways that link your gut and your brain and telling your brain what to crave. They can also tinker with your taste receptors in order to make some foods more appealing than others. In other words, microbes are working behind the scenes to instigate food cravings.

The microbes in question are ones that love sugar and feed on it, so they do everything in their power to compel you to eat sugary foods. If you cave, your cravings for sweets will only intensify.

Many different types of bacterial strains exist in your gut; scientists are still sorting out how each one affects hunger and food cravings. For now, though, the main take-home message from current studies is that if you eat a lot of junk food, this habit fosters the growth of junk-food-craving microbes in your gut. The less you feed them, the less you'll crave junk food.

Here's something else: Success, happiness, even negativity are contagious—they rub off on us from other people. But did you know that cravings and food preferences may be contagious too? When scientists started looking into bacterial-induced eating behaviors, they found that the fecal and oral microbes were more similar among family members who lived together, compared to noncohabiting individuals. If family members in your household have microbes that crave certain foods, you might crave those foods too, because you've got the same microbes. So in other words, you can catch cravings in much the same way that you'd catch a cold or flu.

The good news is that if you build your diet around nutritious foods favored by bacteria that thrive on healthier foods, you will edge out the microbes that are causing you to crave processed foods.

**Cravings Crusher:** Befriend Some Health Food Nuts

We're influenced by other people's eating habits—right down to the microscopic bacteria in their guts. If you hang around or live with people who have healthy eating habits, you might just change the health of your microbiome.

So, you can avoid an unhealthy gut by association! Begin to cook healthy meals for your whole family. The recipes and meal plans in this book will get you started. And enlarge your circle of friends to include those who are interested in eating well.

## WHY YOU MIGHT BE A CHOCOHOLIC

Practically every day, I enjoy some chocolate, especially the antioxidant-rich dark variety. It is so delectable that I think it should be its own food group! You, too, might be a self-proclaimed chocolate lover. However, scientists have discovered that your cravings for chocolate may not even be your own—they may belong to your gut bacteria. Chocoholics have different bacteria in their stomachs compared to people who do not crave chocolate.

A study published in the *Journal of Proteome Research* looked at twenty men, eleven who were categorized as chocolate indifferent and eleven who were chocolate desiring (in other words, chocolate lovers). Researchers analyzed the men's blood and urine for byproducts and found that the metabolic profiles of the two groups were different. One of the most interesting findings was that the urine samples showed different intestinal flora in the two groups. One type of flora feast on chocolate. They grow and ferment it, producing compounds that are anti-inflammatory too. Other types of flora do not exhibit this preference for chocolate. What this means is that if you're a chocoholic, you may be programmed to love chocolate based on the activity and makeup of your gut bacteria.

This isn't necessarily bad news, however. Scientists have studied the benefits of dark chocolate for years, and its health perks are wonderful. From boosting heart health and promoting better blood flow to increasing insulin sensitivity, dark chocolate—in moderation—has an impressive resume.

But one of dark chocolate's real standouts—and quite possibly the reason for its other positive attributes—is that it can nourish your good gut bacteria. In a study published in *Nutrients,* volunteers who consumed antioxidant-rich cocoa for four weeks experienced significant increases in populations of gut rockstars *Bifidobacteria* and *Lactobacillus*. Also, beneficial bacteria can ferment dark chocolate into short-chain fatty acids that fight off harmful bacteria and reinforce the gut lining against invaders.

You don't need much dark chocolate to reap these benefits, however. Indulge in moderation—usually a couple of small squares or ounces—three or four times a week.

## **Cravings Crusher:** How to Manage Pregnancy Food Cravings

Pickles and ice cream. Onions and mustard. A slab of cream cheese slathered with ketchup. While these pairings may give you the yuck factor, if you're pregnant, they can seem like heaven on a plate.

But what's behind the unquenchable longings when you're expecting—and can they be harmful?

Studies have found that pregnancy cravings arise from hormonal fluctuations. These make your sense of smell, taste, and appetite go haywire, and create urges for flavors, textures, and combinations that might seem weird at times.

Other reasons for strange cravings might have to do with nutrients your body wants—for example, craving a bowl of rocky road ice cream might mean your body desires calcium, which is found in ice cream. The process of developing a new life within the womb also bumps up your energy requirements so your body can provide proper fuel for fetal growth. More calories increase blood flow and help in fetal development.

Lastly, some experts think pregnancy cravings represent a normal desire for comfort food because your body is adjusting to a unique physical stress.

Additionally, you may feel hungrier (and thirstier) during breastfeeding, which places an enormous demand on your body and can initiate the desire for food. A pregnant person requires about an extra 300 calories daily, while someone who is breastfeeding needs between 500 to 1000 additional calories each day.

As a doctor, my biggest concern is to make sure pregnancy and breastfeeding food cravings do not replace good nutrition—in other words, don't fill up on the foods you crave while skimping on the nutritious foods your body and baby really need.

Your pregnancy cravings may not pass until your third trimester. So for now, what's the best way to handle them?

- Stock up on healthy snack options like dark chocolate, fruit, nuts, and Greek yogurt.
- Avoid foods that are not healthy during pregnancy: undercooked or raw eggs, alcohol, fish with high mercury

levels (king mackerel, albacore tuna, shark, swordfish, cobia, to name a few), refrigerated smoked seafood, and unpasteurized dairy.

- Try eating or snacking every few hours. This will help stabilize your blood sugar levels and curb cravings before they sideswipe you.
- Stay hydrated (your fluid needs are higher). And note that hunger often masquerades as thirst.
- To emphasize what I said earlier: Concentrate on healthy nutrition during your pregnancy. However, it's perfectly okay to treat yourself once in a while by indulging in common cravings like ice cream.
- Go to www.amymdwellness.com/ pregnancycravingcheatsheet for a tool to help you curb your cravings while pregnant.

All in all, there's no need to be concerned by your weird and wonderful food cravings. Most moms-to-be and new moms crave one food or another during pregnancy and after giving birth.

## MICROBIAL NEUROACTIVES

As part of their metabolic function, microbes break down (metabolize) nutrients. In doing so, they produce by-products called metabolites. Some of these microbial metabolites can mimic hunger or satiety hormones—namely ghrelin, leptin, and peptide YY. Like hormones, metabolites work in sync, signaling us to eat when hungry and stop when full. You'll recall from the earlier discussion of hormones that the more ghrelin being secreted, the more likely you are to overeat. Leptin and peptide YY function in the opposite way, suppressing the appetite and increasing energy levels. Because many gut bacteria can manufacture small peptides that mimic these hormones, they wield significant influence over your appetite.

# PSYCHOBIOTICS AND
# EMOTIONAL EATING

As I mentioned earlier, we all eat emotionally from time to time—when we're down, anxious, or lonely, when we want to comfort ourselves, or even when we're happy or we recall certain food memories from the past, like Grandma's apple pie.

It sounds like something out of a sci-fi movie, but the bacteria within us may very well be influencing not only our cravings, but also our moods to get us to eat what they want. Research shows that your gut microbes manipulate your eating behavior to improve their own health, often at your expense. This can be set into motion by not only triggering cravings for foods that the microbes require but also by depressing your mood until you eat foods that benefit their well-being.

Microbes have the power to do this in surprising ways, both of which affect our emotional health, by manufacturing toxins to make us feel bad or by releasing mood-boosting chemicals to make us feel good.

For example, certain bacteria in the *Clostridium* species generate a substance called propionic acid, which can interfere with your body's production of mood-boosting dopamine and serotonin. On the good side, microbes like *Bifidobacteria* help manufacture butyrate, an anti-inflammatory chemical that prevents gut-generated toxins from entering the brain. Other microbes can synthesize the amino acid tryptophan, a building-block of mood-lifting serotonin.

What's more, certain strains of good bacteria themselves have been shown to act as mood boosters—a major focus of research into psychobiotics. Mood disorders, such as depression and anxiety, have long been associated with an increased likelihood to eat and overeat unhealthy foods.

In a month-long study published in *Brain, Behavior, and Immunity*, healthy volunteers with no previous history of depression were given either probiotics or antidepressants. Those who took the probiotics showed lower cortisol levels and improved moods, similar to what was experienced by participants who took diazepam, a commonly used antianxiety medication. Other similar studies found that pro-biotic therapy can reduce symptoms of depression as well as citalopram (an antidepressant).

Emotional eating also has much to do with the interconnected-ness of the gut and the brain. Most of us are well aware that billions of neurons make up the brain. But did you know that your gut also contains a dense network of neurons? Called the enteric nervous system, this network is in charge of the physiological function of the gastrointestinal tract. In fact, this neuronal network is so active that it has been dubbed the second brain.

In this sense, the gut is an integral part of the central nervous system (the brain and spinal cord) and is connected to it through the gut–brain axis. This term collectively describes the linkage between the gut and the brain via the vagus nerve.

The vagus nerve is quite powerful. Various studies show that stimulating this nerve triggers overeating, whereas blocking it leads to weight loss.

The connection between the gut and the brain is reflected by our language in the way we describe our emotions. We say things like "It's gut wrenching," "That makes me sick," or "I have butterflies in my stomach." Our use of these terms is one result of the number of neurotransmitters produced in the gut, according to a review article published in *Gastroenterology Clinics of North America*. They en-able the nervous system to function and communicate.

All of this suggests that the gut–brain axis affects emotions, and emotions strongly influence food choices, as well as appetite.

Your overall mental health is also affected by psychobiotics. While studying psychobiotics for this book, I ran across a fascinating study from China published in *Science Advances* that illustrated most definitively how much microbes truly control how we think and feel. The research uncovered new evidence that our gut microbes may be related to schizophrenia and mental health. We already know through prior studies that alterations in gut bacteria affect anxiety and depression.

This 2019 study probed the connection between schizophrenia and changes in gut bacteria. Schizophrenia is a hard-to-treat, devastating mental disorder that brings on hallucinations, a fractured sense of reality, and disordered thinking. It is a lifelong condition that can be severely disabling. The findings of this study might lead to more effective ways to treat schizophrenia.

The researchers started out by analyzing fecal samples from sixty-three patients suffering from schizophrenia. Their samples were compared against a control group of sixty-nine people not experiencing schizophenia. Overall, the schizophrenic subjects had less microbial diversity in their microbiome than the healthy controls. The dissimilarities in the gut bacteria between the patients and healthy controls were so obvious, in fact, that the researchers could identify the schizophrenic patients by their stool samples alone. The next phase of the study became even more interesting. The researchers transplanted fecal samples from human schizophrenic patients into healthy, germ-free mice. The same process was also done using healthy human fecal samples to create an effective control group. The mice colonized with the schizophrenic microbiome soon showed behavioral changes that have been associated with mouse models of schizophrenia.

The researchers also analyzed levels of glutamate in mouse brains. Glutamate is a neurotransmitter that does not work normally in schizophrenics. The mice with gut bacteria from the schizophrenic humans exhibited abnormal glutamate in their brains. The gut bacteria appeared to have changed the brain's chemicals. This was an important finding because disruptions in glutamate metabolism have long been strongly hypothesized as an underlying cause of schizophrenia.

So, your gut microbes? As bizarre as it seems, they are very much at work controlling your mental health.

## Cravings Crusher: SOS for PMS Cravings

You likely experience cravings around your menstrual period. That's normal. There are a few causes: the ups and downs of estrogen and progesterone, how these hormones affect your mood, and what they do to your desire for sweets, as well as drop in serotonin, our natural mood booster.

You can circumvent these cravings and boost your mood at the same time by following a few simple suggestions.

Fish for relief with foods high in omega-3 fatty acids (think salmon, tuna, sardines, and other fatty fish). Omega-3s stabilize hormonal fluctuations and mood swings.

Go nuts—Brazil nuts, that is. Anxiety has been associated with a deficiency in the mineral selenium. You can easily fulfill your entire daily selenium requirement by eating three Brazil nuts each day.

Be proactive with probiotics. These foods (yogurt, kombucha, kimchi, and so forth) steady your hormones and keep serotonin on the upswing. Include a couple of servings a day when you have PMS-related cravings.

Go for dark chocolate. It's an antidote to cravings and moodiness—plus enjoyable to eat. Chocolate is also a serotonin booster. Have 1 to 2 ounces daily.

Stay consistent with exercise. It's one of the best ways to lift your mood and relieve PMS symptoms, including cravings.

Follow the 5 steps in this book. Each one is designed to keep hunger and cravings in check—at all stages of your life.

## REBUILD A HEALTHY MICROBIOME IN JUST A FEW DAYS

If you think you're defenseless against the will of your microbes right now, don't worry. You are not. Understand that there are many ways you can manipulate them—simply by tapping into the power of psychobiotics through your food choices, probiotics, and prebiotics.

First, know this: Your gut microbiome regenerates every half hour or so because bacteria have a short life cycle. What you eat now—say for breakfast, lunch, or dinner—will begin to alter the diversity of your microbiome right away and normalize your hunger sensations.

Continue to make good food choices, and you can begin to override your urges and cravings and rebuild your microbiome in just a few days. Let that sink in. You have the power to create immediate improvements in your gut health and diversity. I'll cover this more in the 5-step plan, but here are some psychobiotic strategies you can take now.

## Focus on Fiber

Begin to regenerate your microbiome overnight with just a few good, fiber-filled veggies—although to really make the change stick you'll need to eat these foods several times a week.

Adding fiber is crucial, as well. High-fiber foods are more satiating than low-fiber foods, so you're likely to eat less and stay satisfied longer. Combining protein with high-fiber vegetables fills you up even faster.

For background, dietary fiber is technically the nondigestible parts of plant foods. We don't think of it as a nutrient, but it is—an important one. Unlike the major macronutrients—namely fat, protein, or carbohydrates, which your body breaks down and absorbs—fiber passes relatively intact through your digestive tract and is eliminated from your body.

There are two classifications of fiber: soluble, meaning it dissolves in water, or insoluble, which doesn't dissolve. Top sources of soluble fiber include oats, peas, beans, apples, citrus fruits, carrots, barley, and psyllium. Job one for soluble fiber is to slow digestion so your body has enough time to absorb nutrients from the food you eat.

Whole grains, nuts, beans, legumes, and many veggies, like broccoli, green beans, and potatoes, are rich in insoluble fiber. Because it binds with water as it passes through your digestive tract, insoluble fiber makes the stool softer, thus easing the risk of constipation and protecting your digestive system. Both types of fiber are excellent food sources for the good bacteria in your gut.

Most gut bacteria reside in the distal colon, the last stop in the intestines, so getting high-fiber food there is key. Most of what we eat—namely protein, fats, and many carbs—gets digested prior to reaching the distal colon. Fiber, on the other hand, does not, so the good bacteria can feed on it when it arrives at the distal colon.

What if we don't get enough fiber? The bacteria that love fiber will not thrive, decreasing your gut diversity. Imbalanced gut bacteria and a low-fiber diet lead to the dreaded condition suffered by my patient Robert—dysbiosis. Dysbiosis makes you vulnerable to many serious diseases, including inflammatory bowel disorder, colitis, leaky gut, obesity, diabetes, and other serious chronic conditions.

## Enjoy Prebiotics

The food you feed your friendly gut bugs is as important as the bugs themselves in getting them to grow and colonize. One of the best foods for gut microbes is a type of fiber known as prebiotics. Think of prebiotics as fast food for gut microbes. They feed and encourage the growth of good bacteria. As for hunger and cravings, they help our satiety hormones spring into action.

To increase your intake of prebiotics, you should eat more cellulose fibers, found in the tough parts of vegetables and fruit (think of broccoli stalks, the bottoms of asparagus, kale stems, and orange pulp).

The following foods are also rich in prebiotics:

- Beans and legumes
- Dark chocolate
- Fibrous parts of fruits and vegetables
- Garlic
- Ginger
- Jerusalem artichokes
- Leeks (green and white parts)
- Onions
- Plantains
- Potatoes, yams, sweet potatoes, and other root vegetables

## Add Fermented Foods and Probiotics

For an extra jolt of gut-enriching nutrients, populate your diet with fermented foods. Fermentation is a biochemical magic trick in which yeast turns sugar into alcohol, though many other micro-organisms and foods can ferment as well.

Throughout history, fermented foods occurred serendipitously: honey water accidentally turned into mead, as did grapes to vinegar. But pretty soon, people learned how to ferment foods all by themselves. By 5400 B.C., wine came on the scene, thanks to the ancient Iranians. By 1800 B.C., the Sumerians were brewing beer. By the first century B.C., the Chinese had concocted an early version of what we now know as soy sauce.

Today, fermentation generally uses a starter containing microbes or bacteria naturally present in food to create a different version of a food or change its properties. You probably eat a lot of fermented foods already and don't even realize it, like cheese, olives, or sour cream.

Essentially, the good bacteria in the food or starter begin to break down sugars and starches. This gives off lactic acid, which halts the growth of bad bacteria, so the food doesn't spoil. The food is preserved, plus becomes more nutritious than it was before.

There are some wonderful benefits to adding fermented foods to your diet. Fermented foods are:

*More digestible.* During fermentation, the bacteria predigest the food. As a result, the fermented food is easier on your digestive system.

*Highly nutritious.* The bacteria in fermented foods manufacture extra vitamins and nutrients, such as B vitamins and vitamin K2, as they digest the starches and sugars.

*Packed with probiotics.* Some medical and nutrition authorities report that each ½ cup serving of a fermented food can hold up to 10 trillion probiotic organisms—for this reason, I feel that it is better to obtain probiotics by eating fermented foods rather than relying on dietary supplements.

*Immune system boosters.* Approximately 80 percent of your immune system is headquartered in your gut. Eating fermented foods on a regular basis helps ensure a healthy and diverse gut—and a healthy immune system.

*Cravings controllers.* By supplementing your diet with fermented foods, you can actually control your sweet cravings. How? Fermented foods assist your taste buds in adapting to more bitter or sour flavors, so you're less likely to gravitate to, or crave, sugary foods.

To strengthen and diversify your microbiome, consider trying the following fermented foods and drinks, which are full of ready-made probiotic bacteria.

FERMENTED FOODS
- Kimchi
- Kombucha
- Miso
- Natto
- Sauerkraut
- Tempeh

FERMENTED DAIRY (IF YOU CAN TOLERATE IT)
- Cottage cheese
- Kefir
- Sour cream
- Yogurt

## Aim for a Nutrient-Dense Diet

Remember that a diverse microbiome tends to be a healthy microbiome. A great way to achieve this is through a nutrient-dense diet. What does that mean, exactly?

Nutrient density identifies the amount of nutrients such as vitamins, minerals, and amino acids in a given food, relative to its calories (which are usually low). This term is not to be confused with "energy density." Foods that are energy dense have lots of calories per serving (usually due to added sugar or fat or other detrimental ingredients), while nutrient-dense foods are packed with mostly beneficial nutrients with little or no added sugars or fats that raise calories.

Some foods, like vegetables, have very high nutrient density, while processed foods have low nutrient density and a higher energy density. Think of the difference between 160 calories' worth of potato chips and a plain baked potato, also 160 calories. The baked potato supplies approximately 4 grams of fiber, 950 milligrams of potassium, 17 milligrams of vitamin A, 22 milligrams of vitamin C, and no saturated fat. The potato chips, on the other hand, provide no fiber or vitamins, half the potassium, and 3 grams of saturated fat. The baked potato, therefore, is far more nutrient dense than the caloric equivalent of potato chips.

A nutrient-dense diet is also balanced with an ample supply of protein, fat, and fiber in order for us to feel satisfied. Protein helps regulate leptin and ghrelin, so that we feel comfortably full. Quality fats such as omega-3 fatty acids, and fats from plant sources assist with the production of leptin to signal fullness and slow down our digestion. A high-fiber intake sparks the production of short-chain fatty acids, which also help your body feel full, and creates a diversity of good gut bacteria in your microbiome.

Choose mostly nutrient-dense foods, and you'll take in more nutritious macronutrients, vitamins, minerals, and amino acids that promote good health, and avoid too many processed, energy-dense foods that can lead to overweight or obesity. What's more, a nutrient-dense diet supplies nutritious fuel to all those good microbes that support your health and prevent any one population from taking over too much gut territory. You'll happily discover that your cravings will subside substantially by following a nutrient-dense diet for several months, thanks to a shift in the diversity of your microbiome.

You can expect your gut health to improve fairly quickly once you've increased fiber and prebiotics, populated your diet with fermented foods and probiotics, emphasized a nutrient-dense diet, and decreased common gut wreckers like sugar and junk food. And along with all this, there's more great news: fewer cravings and better hunger control, because you and your gut microbes are working in sync.

# Unlearned Eating: Are You Really Hungry?

WHEN IT COMES TO HUNGER and overeating, Marcy is probably like many of you. She goes to a party on the weekend, and eats lots of chips and dip, sometimes with a few glasses of wine. She goes home feeling guilty and full of regret, and vows to run a few extra miles the next day. The rest of the weekend, Marcy eats like a bird and feels proud of herself.

But this doesn't last too long. She gets so hungry that she just can't stop eating junk food, especially sweets, as if there is about to be some kind of worldwide dessert shortage.

By midweek, Marcy embarks on the next new diet and is careful about what she eats. Although still hungry, she powers through her hunger, feeling full of willpower. But after a particularly grueling day as an ER nurse, Marcy sits on the couch and vegs for hours, which usually means keeping company with a pint of ice cream. She feels completely out of control.

The way Marcy eats and lives offers a habitual glimpse into her life. She's unhappy with it and desperately wants to find a solution.

She asks me: "Why can't I be more consistent and eat healthy more of the time? I feel like I can't stop eating. If I don't get this under control, I'm going to be in real trouble."

If you can relate to Marcy's situation, forget all about diet books, weight-loss programs, even willpower, which ebbs and flows based on what's happening to us and how we feel. There is, however, hope around the corner. These cycles of hunger and overeating can stop—and quickly.

As you have now read, our brain, gut, neurons, and hormones are all connected. Various hunger hormones are secreted into the bloodstream from our gut, signaling the brain that it's time to restock the body's fuel supply. Other hormones put the brakes on eating. Neurons transmit hunger signals back and forth between our brain and gut. Microbes in the gut are commandeering whether we reach for cookies or cauliflower.

Other forces are intertwined in the mix. We see food, we smell it. We might read or think about it. People, places, and things remind us of a good meal. We're further tempted by our constant exposure to highly palatable foods tempting us to eat, eat, and eat some more. There are only so many times that we can resist a platter of freshly baked cookies that pass by before we grab one.

So now that you understand that everything is connected, how can you optimize it? That's the goal, right?

The first step is to realize that the body is an amazing, self-regulatory system. It knows exactly how much food you need and sends all sorts of signals indicating when it's truly hungry and when it's full. When you understand this system—I mean really understand—your whole relationship with food and hunger will change. You will learn, as Marcy did, to stop trying to control your hunger with willpower and stop compensating for unhealthy overeating with equally unhealthy undereating.

The way to end these crazy cycles of hunger, cravings, and overeating is to apply some tactics I collectively call unlearned eating.

WTF is unlearned eating? In a nutshell, it involves:

- Becoming more aware of what real hunger feels like.
- Responding less to external and environmental eating cues.
- Listening to your body and responding to its needs appropriately.
- Modifying eating triggers that work against you.
- Making peace with your body because you have a healthier, happier relationship with food than previously.

Let's take a deeper dive into exactly how unlearning eating works—and how to make it work for you.

## UNLEARNED EATING IS NOT THE SAME AS INTUITIVE EATING

Set forth as a strategy to control hunger, intuitive eating is perhaps something you've heard about. This hot diet buzzword means you listen and respond to internal prompts (stomach growling, low blood sugar, etc.) to eat, instead of external signals (like a food ad or the sight, smell, or taste of delicious-looking foods). In other words, you eat when you're truly hungry, and stop when you're full.

Also, intuitive eating rejects any kind of diet mentality—no type of food is off-limits. Instead, it involves learning to be more mindful of how much to eat and becoming aware of your satiety level and recognizing when to stop eating.

All this sounds good in theory, and I'm not bashing this strategy, but, unfortunately, many people have huge problems with intuitive eating when they start trying to follow it. For example:

- What do you do when you're so bombarded with food advertising that it prods you into eating too much of a lot of foods you don't really need in your diet? This is a big problem in our society, because we live in a world jam-crammed with external cues for eating. Practically everywhere, streets are lined with restaurants, eateries, and fast food joints trying to draw us in, and the media screams with food ads. Even at home we aren't safe from the lure of external cues, since a lot of kitchens are well stocked with food waiting inside the fridge or pantry.

- How about being so overexposed to ultrapalatable processed foods that you have a hard time resisting them? Unlike our ancient ancestors, who had to walk miles to get water, find edible plants, and hunt for animals, we forage at fast food establishments, which are usually a mile or two from our front doors. And, as we talked about earlier, modern foods are combinations of flavors, textures, tastes, and aromas that literally hijack our body's natural system of satiety. In this type of food environment, intuitive eating takes a lot of white-knuckling willpower to resist the lure of sweets, desserts, snacks, fast foods, and other indulgences.
- How do you make sure you're eating important hunger-control and satiety-boosting foods like omega-3 fatty acids, prebiotics and probiotics, various types of fiber, and certain amino acids?
- What happens when stress and emotions send you headlong into a tub of ice cream or a bag of chips?
- What do you do when your coworkers are eating cake for a birthday celebration?
- How do you handle the fact that your parents raised you on pancakes for breakfast every day, and you often miss that way of starting your day?

Intuitive eating doesn't take into account situations like these.

Let me emphasize, too, that we've grown so deaf to what our bodies are communicating that we can't read or interpret our hunger signals—which means attempts to eat intuitively may be an exercise in futility. Toss in factors like boredom, stress, joy, or food memories and things get even more challenging. We don't know when we're hungry or not, or if we're dealing with out-of-control cravings. And sometimes we eat past the state of fullness.

# INTUITIVE EATING IS GOOD BUT UNLEARNED EATING IS BETTER

Your body is designed to be a very skilled communicator, but sometimes it can be easy to misinterpret its cues. Fortunately, you can fix this with unlearned eating.

Eating—whether it's overeating or eating prodded by external stimuli—is a behavior, an action. And behaviors can be unlearned.

Think of behaviors like you would hiking trails through the woods. The more those trails are used, the clearer they are, and the easier they are to navigate from beginning to end without getting lost. But as trails become unused, they get overgrown, and you're less likely to hike them. Over time it becomes increasing unlikely that you will continue hiking them. That behavior becomes a thing of the past.

Likewise, a big part of unlearned eating is to avoid engaging in certain behaviors—like eating when you're bored or eating processed foods. You can unlearn these habits. When you do, you begin to automatically increase satiety, decrease hunger, and control cravings. Along the way, you also make better food choices and gain a feeling of calm, greater energy, and alertness from the foods you eat.

Unlearned eating helps you easily change behaviors that are influencing your consumptive behavior and interfering with your hunger signals. In the following sections are the key tactics involved in unlearned eating.

## Modify Food Memories

Not that long ago, I detoured down the candy aisle at the grocery store, and a bright red package caught my eye—Kit Kat bars, whose wrapper displayed the luscious, chocolaty wafer treat snapped in half.

I had not had a Kit Kat bar in about thirty years, since the days of my favorite childhood holiday, Halloween. So I bought one, unwrapped it, and ate it, delighting in the crunch of the wafery goodness inside my mouth. It tasted as good as it had when I was a little girl.

The memories didn't stop there, however. In seconds, I was transported back in time to the days of going shopping with my dad to buy Kit Kat bars for Halloween, handing them out to trick-or-treaters, and saving a bunch for my dad and me to eat later (it was his favorite candy bar too). Such fond memories! I finished my Kit Kat bar and returned to the present.

We all have our food memories, and they're mostly good ones. The taste, smell, and texture of certain foods can be extremely evocative, recalling memories not just of eating the food itself but also of people and places—the entire context of where you were, who you were with, and what the occasion was.

Food memories are more evocative and powerful than other memories because they involve all five senses. They don't rely on using just your sight, or just your taste or smell, but rather they involve all the senses working together to layer richness and detail into your brain.

But what is it specifically about childhood candy bars and other goodies that makes them stick in our brains when we are adults?

For one thing, food memories are an evolutionary survival mechanism. Back in ancient days, our hunter-gatherer ancestors had to forage through forests and pastures for fruit and vegetables—and more importantly, remember where the trees and plants that bore them were located, as well as recall which ones tasted particularly good.

Because of our ancestry as food seekers, a highly appealing food will push a button in the brain. Eat that food, and the reward centers of your brain are activated, largely due to the neurotransmitter dopamine surging in response to the reward. Also involved is the hippocampus, which solidifies short-term memories into long-term ones. Together, these reward mechanisms are responsible for what drives memory formation in the brain.

To unlearn the behavior of seeking and craving a nostalgic food, get to the bottom of its appeal like I did. Doing so can put you more in control over how you respond to this food. Ask yourself: Where does this craving for a certain food come from? Is it a childhood memory or other experience that made the food so appealing?

Once you have a better understanding of your neural pathways, use this knowledge to prepare for situations that involve food, know what triggers you, and make listening to your body a priority. Pause and tell yourself, "Yeah, I really could go for that candy bar, and I could get it out of the vending machine right now." But before you do, think about the consequences: cravings for more sweets, more hunger, blood sugar crash, inflammation, and so forth. (I cover this more in Chapter 6.)

It's fine to reminisce about the pleasant memories of people and places from the past, but don't make food the focus of the memory.

## Recognize True Hunger Versus Boredom

Sometimes we have idle moments and simply feel bored. You might wander into the kitchen to see if there is anything to eat to relieve your boredom. You open the fridge, seeking something to munch on. If nothing looks appealing, you move on to the pantry to find a food that doesn't take a lot of time or effort to fix—something you can grab and go.

Are you truly hungry? Not really. You're just looking for something to do.

To unlearn this behavior, figure out some activities to occupy your time and engage your mind. Read. Call a friend. Work on a fun home project. Cross something off your to-do list. A lot of times your feeling of hunger will pass when you focus on something besides food and eating.

**Cravings Crusher:** Lose Your Taste for Sweets in Thirty Days

Sugar can be highly addictive and a diet wrecker. I am often asked: "Can I lose my taste for sugar?"

A great question! Let's look at it scientifically. A study published in 2015 in *The American Journal of Clinical Nutrition* set out to determine what it takes to diminish your taste for sugar. The participants were divided into two groups. One group was instructed to eat a low-sugar diet for three months; the second group served as the control and did not adjust their sugar intake.

Each month of the study, the participants were brought in, fed sweetened pudding, and asked to rate the sweetness of that dessert. During the first month, the low-sugar group and the control group reported the same ratings of sweetness. By the second month, however, the ratings started to change. The low-sugar group found the pudding to be intensely sweet; the control group did not.

After just one month on a low-sugar diet, those participants' taste buds had become more sensitive to sugar. They thought the pudding was too sweet and liked it less.

For those of you with a sweet tooth, this means that after you ease back on eating sugar for awhile, it loses its allure. Sweet foods taste too sweet—and you don't crave them as much, so you don't eat them as often, if at all. And, of course, the less sugar you take in the greater your chance of losing weight or maintaining an ideal weight.

The number-one message here is that you can train your taste buds to dislike intense sweetness, but to get there you need to cut back or even avoid sugar for at least one month, although for some people, it might take longer. Everyone is different, but the point is that you can unlearn your sugar habit.

## Distinguish Between Thirst and Hunger

Many years ago, I learned that when we feel really hungry, thirst might be masquerading as hunger. Our body isn't hungry—it's thirsty. Nonetheless, we mistake that thirst for hunger, and we dive into some food instead. Eating doesn't satisfy the thirst, so we eat more and we might gain weight as a result.

What exactly is going on?

The same satiety centers that beg for food sometimes want to quench thirst rather than eat. As with hunger, thirst can be activated by neurons, hormones in the gut, and even dopamine (no wonder we find water so rewarding when thirsty!). Or thirst could be a physiological response to a meal. Eating food temporarily thickens your blood, and your body senses the need to dilute it.

So—are you actually hungry? No, you're thirsty.

Try this: when feeling hungry, drink a glass or two of water first, to see if that's really what your body wants.

To promote drink-enough-water behavior, stay hydrated throughout the day, too. Keep a glass or bottle (non-BPA plastic, glass, or stainless steel) of water with you at all times. I also suggest drinking an 8-ounce glass of water every morning and keeping a glass by your bed at night. Drink water warm too—it takes less time to digest and stimulates digestion while detoxing your system and aiding food through the digestive tract. Drinking warm water is one of the best actions you can take for your health and to help regulate your hunger.

If not drinking enough water is a bad habit you have, these suggestions, practiced daily, will help you unlearn it.

## Change Your Diet to Promote Satiety

This one is a biggie, and what I've built my 5-step plan around. Ironically, what you put in your mouth is going to be the most important predictor of how you manage hunger, cravings, and satiety.

Of course, I'm on this soapbox a lot, but it's a soapbox worth jumping on, over and over. If we consistently eat a standard low-nutrient, low-fiber diet, we're going to get hungry not long after eating. Not good—true hunger doesn't kick in so early after a meal.

So we must modify our diet to naturally promote satiety and curb hunger. Eating a nutrient-rich diet with lots of fresh plant foods will accomplish this, plus better meet the nutrient needs of our body.

It also boosts our fiber. Fiber may not be the sexiest nutrient around, but it sure works miracles for satiety, hunger control, and overall digestion—especially prebiotic fiber, which feeds our good bacteria and starves the bad, junk-food craving bacteria. Just another reason to eat our fruits and veggies.

Most Americans consume less than 20 grams of fiber a day—they just aren't eating enough of this satiating, digestive-health-supporting nutrient. To unlearn this habit, consume at least one high-fiber plant-based food like beans, whole grains, fruits, and greens at each meal, and you'll feel naturally full and less hungry. Mix up your menu too. Growing research shows that the more variety you have in your plant intake, the more diverse (thus healthy) the bacteria in your gut.

Once you restore nutritional integrity to your diet—and unlearn the habit of eating processed food—your hunger will stabilize and your cravings will dissipate. In an environment of healthy food choices, all the neuronal, hormonal, and psychobiotic factors align and are in sync. You'll then be more tuned into your body's messages on exactly how much food you need at a meal in order to maintain a healthy weight and enjoy long-term health.

## Hunger Hack: High-Water Foods

Feeling hungry too much of the time? In addition to high-fiber foods, protein, and healthy fats (all known to boost satiety), include foods high in water. They help fill your stomach too.

Here's my A-list of nutrient-dense foods that are 90 percent water or more—and will help increase satiety:

*Fruits*
Cantaloupe
Cranberries
Grapefruit
Orange
Peach
Pineapple
Raspberries
Watermelon

*Vegetables*
Celery
Cucumber
Green cabbage
Lettuce
Radishes

Tomato

Zucchini

*Other Foods*

Broths

Clear soups

Try to prioritize your food choices around nutrient-packed, high-fiber, high-water-content foods, and you'll effortlessly get your hunger under control—without having to try to rely on willpower—and protect your precious health in the process.

## Tune into Your Bodyset

You've probably heard a lot about mindset, the collection of beliefs that shapes how you make sense of the world and yourself. Changing your mindset can influence how you think, feel, and behave in any given situation.

But have you ever thought about changing your bodyset?

Bodyset is an awareness of your body's sensations and messages, including hunger, your energy levels, moods, and needs, even the desire to go to the bathroom. Some messages are positive, and some are uncomfortable, but the message itself is neither good nor bad. The messages are always neutral; they are simply pieces of information being sent to you.

Listening to your own body's hunger cues is a valuable component of unlearned eating and making peace with food. As I've said, in today's hectic, on-the-go world, it can be challenging to get in tune with your body's cues because we're so easily distracted by our emotions, factors in our environment, or even social situations. Therefore, we start losing the ability to recognize when we are feeling true hunger or if we're just bored, lonely, or depressed. We're out of touch with our hunger and fullness signals, which makes it easy to undereat or overeat.

Although they are very individualized, here are several common signs—true hunger cues—that it is time to eat:

- Is your stomach: rumbling, growling, or feeling empty?
- Do you feel dizzy, faint, or shaky?
- Do you have a headache?
- Are you having difficulty focusing?
- Are you tired or low on energy?
- What about your mood: Are you irritable or cranky?

It is important to understand these signs of physical hunger because you don't want to get overly hungry and start overeating later.

Also, learning how to tell the difference between the physical need to eat and the mental desire to eat is crucial to your long-term success. That doesn't mean you will ignore feelings of hunger forever, but only until you've learned to recognize the real deal.

Besides identifying your true hunger signals, having a positive bodyset and the awareness that comes with it helps you:

- Become more relaxed and at peace with your body.
- Obtain better health by choosing a nutrient-rich diet, getting more sleep, prioritizing alone time or intimate bonding, remembering to relax, practicing better self-care, or not being wrapped up in habits that aren't serving you.
- Create a stronger self-image, because you like who you are, how you look, and how you feel in your own skin.

## Hunger Hack: Avoid Emotional Eating—the Raw Veggie Test

All of us are going about the day when we feel the desire to eat set in. We might be physically hungry, or we need relief from stress, boredom, or some other uncomfortable emotion.

I suggest the Raw Veggie Test to differentiate between true physical hunger and emotionally driven hunger. To use the test, ask yourself if you would eat a bowl of chopped broccoli. If so, you're physically hungry. Go ahead and have a meal. If you answered no, you're emotionally hungry. You're not really hungry for food. You're hungry for something to self-soothe you when under stress or feeling uncomfortable emotions.

The idea behind this test is to show that when we're physically hungry, any food can satisfy that hunger. If only specific foods will curb the hunger, the underlying reason for the hunger is not physical hunger; it's emotional.

## THE REAL DEAL: YOU ARE GENUINELY HUNGRY

If you've already tried a bunch of my hunger hacks and cravings crushers and you still feel hungry, that's okay! Maybe you are physically hungry. Maybe your body is saying, "Feed me!" Maybe it's calling out for certain nutrients to keep you functioning and healthy, or it desires a combo of protein and fiber to stabilize your blood sugar.

I probably don't need to say this, but here goes: Give your body what it truly wants. If you grab something highly processed or super sweet, you'll temporarily fool your body into thinking that's what it wants. But the body isn't easily so tricked for long. You might be hungry again shortly afterward. There just aren't that many nutrients your body can squeeze out of a cupcake, a candy bar, or potato chips to satisfy your hunger needs.

In the 5 steps that follow in Part II, I explain the specifics of how to live and eat so that you don't have to fight off cravings and hunger based on external, environmental, or emotional cues. I promise that I don't want you to go hungry and deny yourself food. Your body will receive the right amount of nutrients to effortlessly manage all the forces engaged in hunger. No longer will you have to fight addictive drives or struggle to eat less and less. You'll eat and live to nourish your body without uncontrollable and frequent food cravings.

Nothing in the 5 steps says that you should only ever eat for nutrition—food and pleasure go hand in hand and it would be a sad state of affairs to eat only when our stomachs grumbled. Healthy eating, without cravings or wild swings of hunger, is all about balance. Give yourself a little leeway. If it's your birthday, enjoy a slice of cake with a smile. With balance, you'll be much more likely to stick to the plan for the rest of your life.

# Part II

5 Steps to Freedom from
Hunger and Cravings

# 5

## Step 1: Replenish

WHAT IF I TOLD YOU true changes in your health and weight come from eating more, not less. And I mean eating more of the foods that satisfy you."

These words caused quite a stir during a nutrition seminar I presented via Zoom to a large group of high-functioning individuals working at a multinational investment company. Since the pandemic started, I have conducted more than twenty-five virtual seminars, so I know that it can be tough to keep attendees engaged—but I did it!

The expressions on their faces were mixed: wide eyes, gaping mouths, raised, quizzical eyebrows. These folks were definitely interested.

I went on to explain that the best diet is one in which we do not count calories or macros, but simply add in, and prioritize, foods that promote feelings of fullness and satisfaction. When we do this, we zap cravings and uncontrollable hunger, we shed our diet obsession, we lose weight effortlessly (if that's our goal), and we get healthy.

I emphasized that my approach flies in the face of conventional diet advice—which tells you to slash calories, cut carbs, and toss out certain food groups. Instead, I prescribe eating nutrient-dense foods that make you feel satisfied. Most other diets overlook this key satiety factor and don't help you get in touch with your body's own hunger cues.

After my seminar, several people reached out to me for further help. One was Terri, an executive with an investment banking and wealth management firm. She had an intense schedule, with long hours—and little time to restructure her current eating habits. Terri tended to be a grab-and-go eater, frequently picking up food on her way to work and on her way home. She confessed that she felt ravenous a lot of the time and had developed unhealthy cravings for fast foods.

Terri needed a way to establish healthier eating habits, not only in the short-term, but for life. I gave her a list of my Super Six nutrients (which I explain in the next section) to add to her current diet, with instructions to not eliminate any foods that she already ate, but to also eat one food from each of the six categories every day. I had her focus on consuming plenty of healthy fats such as olive oil, sources of lean protein, fresh vegetables and fruits like avocados, and specific dairy products such as yogurt—without resorting to extremes. I explained that if she did this, she'd begin to feel incredibly satisfied and should not have the need or desire for large amounts of unhealthy foods.

Terri worked with me on her revamped diet for a couple of months. Over six weeks, she noticed that her cravings had started to wane. No longer did she have to endure her usual four-o'clock slump, in which she craved something sweet or salty to keep her awake along with coffee. Even her energy levels were higher throughout the day. Gradually, the healthy choices she made edged out the less healthy ones, and she loved that she could still enjoy some of her favorites in moderation, like an occasional glass of wine.

Terri got it—she learned to eat for satiety—which is so much easier and enjoyable than trying to diet on willpower alone.

# THE SUPER SIX

Unlike every other diet you've been on, my plan does not lecture on what you can't eat but rather focuses on target nutrients, or what I call the Super Six, that you add to your diet every day.

The essence of this strategy is to replenish: you fill your diet with more of what you can eat (nutrient-dense foods) and eat fewer processed foods and other less healthy choices. This way of eating is based on consuming many delicious whole foods that can help you reduce your appetite and cravings and improve satiety. Put another way, you have the freedom to choose healthy foods that promote feelings of fullness and satisfaction.

To replenish, make sure you incorporate the following essential hunger tamers every day.

## 1. Glucosinolates

Glucosinolates are good-for-you constituents of plant foods, primarily cruciferous vegetables. These are veggies like broccoli, cabbage, Brussels sprouts, and kale, all very popular vegetables both for their health benefits as well as their versatility in recipes.

Because these vegetables are so fiber- and nutrient-loaded, they tend to be more satisfying than high-carb foods. Plus, they can reduce overeating in the short and long term to support weight loss. They also offer amazing perks when it comes to guarding against serious illnesses, including cancer.

So if these are the sort of veggies you turn your nose up at, be careful! You might be missing out on some seriously important nutrition.

When you eat these veggies, their glucosinolates are broken down by microbes into compounds called metabolites. Metabolites halt inflammation, accelerate your metabolism, and set in motion enzymatic reactions to guard your cells from damage (you'll recall from Chapter 3 that metabolites also mimic hunger or satiety hormones). Glucosinolates also work like natural antibiotics to help ward off bacterial, viral, and fungal infections in the body.

The most common glucosinolate-containing vegetables found on grocery store shelves are:

Arugula
Bok choy
Broccoli
Broccoflower
Broccolini
Brussels sprouts
Cabbage
Cauliflower
Collard greens
Horseradish
Kale
Mustard greens
Radishes
Rutabaga
Turnip
Watercress

## 2. Polyphenols

I was raised in a culture that emphasized Ayurvedic medicine, one of the world's oldest holistic (whole-body) healing systems. Part of it focuses on nutrition and special healing diets. Many of the foods commonly used in the Ayurvedic diet tradition are rich in polyphenols, beneficial organic compounds found in various foods, particularly fruits and vegetables.

Dozens of polyphenol compounds exist naturally in foods, and each of them has a unique impact on human health. When I was growing up, for example, high-polyphenol foods like cloves were used to heal digestive problems, protect the brain, and enhance metabolism. Other foods rich in polyphenols and used in Ayurveda medicine include berries, pomegranates, leafy greens, nuts, and many different kinds of herbs.

Most of us know about antioxidants and how important they are for clearing our bloodstream and neural pathways of toxins we accumulate during the day. Polyphenols are a subset of antioxidants, and they have an array of effects on the body when included in your diet. Some polyphenols keep your skin looking healthy, while others help to promote good gut health, giving your immune system a boost.

Polyphenols are key for controlling hunger, appetite, and cravings.

For one thing, they support the growth of good bacteria, while combating bad bacteria. This builds gut diversity, which helps normalize hunger and appetite. Additionally, polyphenols promote the secretion of satiety hormones by cells in the gut.

Polyphenols can also reduce and control your blood sugar levels—which helps with hunger and cravings. They also assist in churning out insulin, the hormone that signals your body to use glucose efficiently. This beneficial action can help prevent insulin resistance—that dreaded condition in which your body doesn't respond properly to the hormone.

If you want to change your diet and start eating more nutritiously, increasing your intake of polyphenols is an excellent way to start. Foods high in polyphenols include:

Avocadoes
Berries, all types
Broccoli
Cherries
Chili peppers
Citrus fruits
Coffee
Flaxseeds
Dark chocolate
Garlic
Legumes
Mangoes
Nuts, all varieties

Olives

Onions

Oregano, as well as many other herbs and spices (choose
    organic if you can in order to avoid pesticide residue)

Pumpkin

Spinach

Tea, all types especially green tea

## Cravings Crusher: The Peppermint Sniff Remedy

Rich in polyphenols, peppermint can defuse cravings
when you sniff it, and you might end up not grabbing a
particular treat.

That's what happened when subjects inhaled a peppermint
scent throughout the day in a 2008 study from Wheeling
Jesuit University in West Virginia published in the journal
*Appetite*. They whiffed the peppermint aroma every two hours
over a five-day period. Each time, they ended up eating about
360 fewer calories daily compared to days when they didn't
inhale peppermint.

Why did the peppermint scent quash cravings so
powerfully? Scientists haven't figured out the answer yet, but
it may have something to do with the fact that the smell of
peppermint is known to boost mood. A better mood might
dampen your desire for high-calorie comfort foods, resulting
in your being able to fend off food cravings.

There are a few ways to experience the benefits of
peppermint yourself: Keep some sprigs of fresh peppermint
nearby, brew peppermint tea, or dab a few drops of
peppermint essential oil on a cotton ball, then enjoy deep
whiffs periodically throughout the day. Diffusing peppermint
essential oil into the air may also do the trick. Popular now,
too, are aromatherapy necklaces that diffuse essential oils into
the air around you all day long.

### 3. Appetite-Suppressing Amino Acids

We've talked about how eating protein at meals can fill you up faster than eating simple carbs like bread and pasta. One of the main reasons for this benefit is the amino acids found in proteins. Maybe you've read about amino acids in a fitness magazine, seen them in the supplement aisle of your pharmacy, or heard about them in an ad.

But what exactly do they do?

In simple terms, amino acids are the building blocks of protein, and they support many of your body's most vital functions, ranging from digesting food to building muscle to helping the body burn fat.

They are also natural appetite suppressants. In fact, a 2009 review published in *The American Journal of Clinical Nutrition* reported that protein and amino acids are more powerful than carbohydrates and fat in promoting short-term satiety in animals and humans. Ingesting amino acids will impart the sensation of feeling full and help you stop overeating.

Certain amino acids satisfy hunger more quickly than others, say reports published in *Nutrients* and other journals. A closer look at these amino acids and their food sources follows.

*Arginine and lysine.* According to researchers at the University of Warwick in England, foods that are high in arginine and lysine can powerfully control your appetite. Their 2017 study found that brain cells called tanycytes are involved in appetite control. After exposing tanycytes from the brain tissue of mice to these two amino acids, the researchers discovered that these cells released satiety signals to the brain within just thirty seconds! The finding suggests that eating more of the amino acids lysine and arginine can flick off your hunger switch. This study was published in the journal *Molecular Metabolism*.

Animal and plant sources of foods high in these aminos include:

Almonds
Apricots
Avocadoes

Beef
Chicken
Lentils
Plums
Pork

*Phenylalanine.* Of all amino acids, this one appears to be the most potent appetite suppressant. It reduces appetite by controlling the release of cholecystokinin, a hormone of the intestines that sends fullness signals to the brain after eating. It also causes the digestion process to perform at a slower pace; this also creates a natural decrease in your appetite.

Foods high in phenylalanine include:

Beans
Beef
Chicken
Fish
Milk
Nuts
Seeds
Sweet potatoes
Tofu
Whole grains

*Tyrosine.* Tyrosine works as an appetite suppressant but on a mild level, because it also triggers cholecystokinin production. What's more, tyrosine stimulates the production of certain hormones that are involved in accelerating the metabolism and fat burning. Tyrosine is also the main building block of dopamine, which plays a role in hunger and cravings (see "Dopamine-Support Foods" on page 84). A lack of tyrosine can result in emotional overeating and depression.

Foods rich in tyrosine include:

Banana
Beans and lentils

Cheese
Eggs
Fish
Pork
Poultry
Prunes
Seeds
Spirulina

*Tryptophan.* This amino acid suppresses the appetite both indirectly and directly. Directly—by elevating the level of your serotonin. Serotonin, in turn, sends a signal to your hypothalamus initiating the sense of being full, decreasing your appetite. Tryptophan functions indirectly like phenylalanine by sending a signal to the intestines to release cholecystokinin to the blood, making you feel full.

Tryptophan-rich foods include:

Beans
Beef
Eggs
Milk
Nuts
Oatmeal
Pork
Poultry
Seeds
Tofu

*Leucine.* This amino acid is beneficial in maintaining lean muscle mass. It also triggers your sense of being full. The effects of this amino acid on weight loss are very powerful. In a study published in *Diabetes, Metabolic Syndrome, and Obesity: Targets and Therapy,* participants lost twice as much weight when taking a leucine supplement, along with vitamin B6, compared to those who took a placebo.

Foods high in leucine include:

Beef
Cottage cheese
Eggs
Lentils
Hemp seeds
Navy beans
Oatmeal
Peanuts
Pork
Pumpkin seeds
Sesame seeds
Spirulina
Tuna

## 4. Dopamine-Support Foods

Intertwined with hunger and satiety hormones are neurotransmitters, including dopamine. Remember, dopamine stimulates the reward and pleasure centers in the brain, which can impact both mood and food intake. Dopamine is often called the motivator molecule because it is responsible for sending signals to your brain to drive behavior.

While it is true that foods both high in sugar and fat (junk food) spike dopamine levels, there's a rebound effect. Those same foods can bump up your appetite, lead to overeating, and possibly cause weight gain over the long haul.

So are there foods that can boost dopamine, but without that rebound effect? Yes—protein!

This fact first came to light in a 2014 issue of *Nutrition Journal*, in which researchers compared the satiety effects from high-protein breakfasts (containing 35 grams of high-quality animal protein) versus normal-protein breakfasts (13 grams) or breakfast skipping in overweight and obese teenage girls. The high-protein breakfast worked best at curbing postmeal cravings and boosting dopamine levels.

This study was the first to show that dopamine surges after you eat protein. As I noted above, protein contains amino acids, several of which are the building blocks of dopamine. Thus, eating more protein is a healthier way to increase dopamine production.

So, what exactly should you eat if you want to raise your dopamine levels? Among the best choices are foods that are rich in tyrosine, the amino acid building block of dopamine. Think chicken, fish, and lean beef. For animal proteins, choose organic, grass-fed, hormone-free, and antibiotic-free, and, for fish, wild-caught as much as possible.

Generally, I think our society eats too much animal protein. I advise that my patients adhere to a plant-based diet for 90 percent of the time. Plant foods that give a big dopamine boost include nuts and seeds, especially raw almonds, pumpkin seeds, walnuts, and chia and hemp seeds.

Foods rich in sulfur compounds also help release dopamine. So, add some collards, Brussels sprouts, cabbage, cauliflower, kale, onions, garlic, and scallions into your diet.

Folate foods are also hailed as foods that aid dopamine production. So, you'll certainly want to get a healthy handful of leafy greens, broccoli, cauliflower, chickpeas, black beans, papaya, and lentils into your meals.

Dark chocolate is also a healthy snack for anyone looking for foods that boost dopamine levels. Not only will this mood-boosting superfood increase dopamine levels but it'll also help boost serotonin as well.

Grab a handful of blueberries and strawberries the next time you need some motivation. These delicious berries are rich in antioxidants that have been shown to protect major parts of the brain that control dopamine production.

## 5. Omega-3 Fatty Acids

These awesome fats should be in your diet routinely because they are part of every cell in your body. They also help strengthen your immune system, support the health of your lungs and blood vessels, and help manufacture hormones.

As we've seen, appetite is regulated by complex neural and hormonal mechanisms that try to maintain homeostasis (aka keep things the same) in the body. Now, growing research has underscored how powerfully these fats support that regulatory system by boosting satiety. In a study published in *Appetite,* obese and overweight individuals felt full sooner during meals containing omega-3 fats than later.

A study reported in the *European Journal of Clinical Nutrition* sheds light on this. It turns out that omega-3 fats boost leptin levels in obese subjects. Leptin is the I'm-full hormone. The same study noted that these powerful fats increase levels of adiponectin, a hormone assigned the jobs of regulating glucose levels and breaking down fat into fatty acids to be used as fuel.

Omega-3 fatty acids suppress appetite in another way—by stimulating the release of the gut and satiety hormone cholecystokinin.

What does all this mean? Omega-3 fats are potent, natural appetite tamers!

Foods high in omega-3 fatty acids include:

Algae oil (this is one of the best sources of vegan omega-3 DHA
    and my preferred omega-3 fat)
Eggs fortified with omega-3s
Fish (especially anchovies, herring, lake trout, salmon, and
    sardines). Fish can contain an excessive amount of mercury,
    pesticide residues, and other toxins, depending on their
    source. Make sure you choose wild caught and organic as
    much as possible.
Nuts and seeds (flaxseeds, walnuts, nut butters, and chia seeds)
Other plant sources such as spirulina, spinach, red lentils, navy beans
Plant oils (flaxseed oil and canola oil). Cold-pressed oils are preferred.

## 6. All Forms of Fiber

I hope you're not getting tired of hearing about fiber (I'll be brief here!), but it is ultra-important for hunger regulation and satiety. It's best to eat the following forms of fiber every day.

Soluble fiber dissolves in water and turns into a gel-like substance during digestion, which helps slow down the process and make you feel full. The best sources of soluble fiber are:

Apples
Avocado
Black beans
Broccoli
Sweet potatoes

Insoluble fiber does not break down in the digestive system but works to help move food through the stomach and intestines. It's like a vacuum for your digestive system. The best sources are:

Bran
Cauliflower
Green beans
Nuts
Whole grains

Prebiotic fiber encourages the growth of good bacteria (probiotics) in your gut—which ultimately helps dampen cravings for sugar and keeps your hunger in check.

The top sources are:

Asparagus
*Banana
Chicory root
*Garlic
Jerusalem artichoke
*Leek
*Onion
Virtually any vegetable
*Wheat

Note that I placed an asterisk next to five prebiotic foods. I'm singling them out for honorable mention because they contain natural compounds called inulin-type fructans, a special type of prebiotic fiber that confers health benefits through alterations in the microbiome. In a 2019 study published in *The American Journal of*

*Clinical Nutrition,* volunteers who increased these fibers in their diets experienced greater satiety and fewer urges to eat sweet, salty, and fatty foods, and actually craved inulin-rich vegetables. Just more reasons to eat prebiotic fiber!

## Add in Fermented Foods

Fermented foods are definitely a healthy food choice for you, as we talked about earlier. They contain probiotic compounds that provide protection to the digestive system. A Stanford study confirmed this amazing fact, too, noting that a diet rich in fermented foods creates a diverse microbiome and reduces chronic inflammation. This study is an early example of how one simple change in your diet can alter your microbiome for the better. It was published in the journal *Cell.*

Yogurt—one of the giants among fermented foods—has been well studied for its effect on satiety. A 2015 report in *Nutrition Reviews* noted that drinking milk and eating yogurt increases the circulating concentration of two important appetite-suppressing hormones: glucagon-like peptide-1 (GLP-1) and peptide YY (PPY).

Produced in the gut, GLP-1 helps regulate your appetite, especially after eating. Because GLP-1 reduces hunger after a meal, if your body releases less of this hormone, you may overeat.

Be careful with diets, too. Dieting has been linked to a decrease in GLP-1. When levels of this hormone fall, your appetite may increase, and you might regain any lost pounds. This situation is yet another reason why traditional diets don't work well.

PPY is another hormone that regulates hunger and sidetracks the desire to eat. For anyone who struggles with excessive hunger, it can be very beneficial to trigger these hormones naturally. Pass the yogurt, please!

I've always tried to include yogurt and fermented foods in my diet, based on what we know about the health benefits of probiotics. Plus, these foods have merits: sauerkraut and kimchi are made from vegetables, which are super good for you, and yogurt is an excellent source of protein. I enjoy eating them; they're easy to find and include in my diet.

It's time for you to get serious and eat fermented foods on a regular basis. Here's a list of the most common fermented foods that you can add to your diet.

Cheeses
Cottage cheese
Kefir
Kimchi
Kombucha, low sugar (fermented tea)
Miso
Olives
Pickles
Sauerkraut
Tempeh
Yogurt

## Hunger Hack: Eat Walnuts, Stay Full

For some time now, scientists have known that eating walnuts makes you feel full. But why? A study conducted by scientists at the Harvard-affiliated Beth Israel Deaconess Medical Center (BIDMC) uncovered what's actually going on in the brain to make this happen.

The researchers recruited ten obese volunteers to live at BIDMC's Clinical Research Center for two five-day sessions. During one of those sessions, the volunteers drank smoothies each day—smoothies that contained 48 grams of walnuts (the daily recommended serving, according to the American Diabetes Association).

During the other session, the volunteers drank a placebo smoothie that was nutritionally comparable to the other smoothie and tasted the same, but was blended without walnuts. The volunteers weren't told which smoothies they were receiving during which session.

Here's what happened: The volunteers reported that they felt less hungry during the week that they drank the walnut smoothies (this did not happen when they had the placebo smoothies). MRI scans taken on the fifth day of each session gave the research team a clear picture as to why. They found that consuming walnuts activates an area in the brain called the right insula, which is associated with regulating hunger and cravings. Basically, eating walnuts changes brain activity to lessen food cravings. This study was published in *Diabetes, Obesity, and Metabolism* in 2018.

Walnuts, anyone?

## REPLENISH AND SUPERCHARGE YOUR DIET WITH THE SUPER SIX

Every day, the goal is to obtain at least one food from each of the six categories. Be sure to check out the recipes in Chapter 11 because they will help you eat foods from the Super Six. Eating more Super Six nutrients is the first step toward replenishing your body and normalizing your hunger cues.

In addition, here are some ways to enjoy these hunger tamers and maximize their benefits:

- Slice some red cabbage into a salad for added nutrition, fiber, and color.
- Roast Brussels sprouts in a little olive oil. Eat them as a side dish, or chill and toss them into a salad.
- Enjoy fresh cole slaw as a side dish.

- Quickly stir-fry bok choy or mustard greens to add to Asian dishes.
- Dip raw broccoli, radishes, and cauliflower in hummus or a yogurt dip.
- Add high-polyphenol fruits and vegetables to your smoothies.
- Spice your eggs and other dishes with herbs.
- Make stir-frys and salads with high-polyphenol veggies.
- Sprinkle whole-grain cereals with various types of seeds.
- Drink a cup of tea or coffee or kombucha with meals for an extra polyphenol or probiotic punch.
- Instead of having sweets for dessert after dinner, choose a few pieces of dark chocolate or a bowl of berries with a dollop of yogurt.
- Sprinkle chia seeds on whole-grain cereal or yogurt in the morning.
- Have smoked salmon on a salad or bake some nut-crusted fish fillets for dinner.
- Sprinkle walnuts on a salad or over baked chicken for dinner.
- Add flaxseeds to pancake batter or use flaxseed oil as a base for salad dressings.
- Prepare a tuna salad with an omega-3-packed oil like flaxseed instead of mayonnaise for a fast lunch.
- Toss some frozen avocado chunks into your smoothie or mash avocados for a veggie dip. Better yet, spoon avocado over fish for an omega-3 two-fer.
- Of course, try as many of my recipes as possible. They're all hunger tamers!

Start to really live Step 1 by centering your food choices on those listed here. You'll automatically clean up your diet with more hunger tamers and fewer processed foods and sweets. I recommend that you follow the meal plans on pages 158–162, too. They will help you get in the swing of my program, and pretty soon, eating and living this way will become a positive, second-nature habit.

# 6

## Step 2: Rewire

I AM SO ADDICTED TO SUGAR."

Obviously distressed, Tina, a 36-year-old programmer, spilled her story to me about craving sugar: Eating an entire pint of ice cream. Snagging leftover cookies from her kids' plates. Digging into a stash of M&Ms at work. These situations were common for her.

"My feelings of shame and failure are overwhelming. I feel almost helpless around sugar. I'm pretty tuned into my body, and I know all this is at the root of my GI troubles and my poor relationship with food. But I'm just addicted."

She continued, "Not a day goes by when I don't plan to quit sweets. But then three o'clock rolls around, and here I go again. I try so hard, but when I fail, I'm so embarrassed. I don't want to live like this. I want to take control."

Tina felt like sugar owned her. It had a stranglehold over her life.

Can you relate? I know I can. There was a time during my fellowship at Columbia Presbyterian when every day I would treat myself to a Starbucks drink—usually a peppermint mocha or an iced caramel macchiato. Each time, I'd tell myself that it was just a treat for that day. But then the very next day, I'd find myself getting that treat again. I look back on the sugar content in those drinks, and I can't believe that I had been gulping down 200 percent of my daily allowance of sugar in ONE beverage!

What I didn't realize at the time, nor did Tina, is that sugar can affect the brain much like cocaine does (as you know from Chapter 1), triggering the same reward centers that this dangerous drug does. It's no surprise, then, that many people feel like they're hooked on sugar, and they can't stop at just one serving of the sugary food. Complicating matters is that sugar in foods takes your blood sugar on a roller coaster ride that brings you right back to where you started so you grab even more of the food. It's a terrible ride, and I have seen many people struggle with it.

But are food addictions, including a sugar addiction like Tina's, real? I think so.

Science backs up my opinion. In animal and human studies, sugar has been found to produce many drug-like effects: bingeing, cravings, tolerance, withdrawal, rewards, and highs. Scientists have added to this research by finding that continuous exposure to hyperpalatables—those sugary/fatty/salty foods with perfect bliss points—rewires the brain's reward center so that we crave more and more of the addicting food.

Food addictions are fairly widespread, too. A 2013 report in *PLOS One* assessed the prevalence of food addiction in 652 men and women using an instrument known as the Yale Food Addiction Scale. Researchers found that:

- Approximately one in twenty people (5 percent of the general population) met the criteria for food addiction.
- A large number of people are almost addicted, meaning they did not meet all the criteria for food addiction but demonstrated a strong association between food and addictive behavior.
- Those with a true food addiction were heavier and had higher body fat percentages than those without such addictions.
- Women were more prone to food addictions than men.

In a nutshell, whether it's a fast-food cheeseburger with fries or sugar-laced snack cakes, any highly palatable processed food can rewire the brain's reward mechanism so that we crave more and more of it much the same way people crave drugs or alcohol.

BUT wait—I have a secret to share with you. Well, it's not a secret in the world of neuroscience, but it is a secret to all of us who are trying to deal with hunger and cravings. We've been in the dark because no one has taught us much about the connection between food and the brain. The secret: it is entirely possible to rewire your brain so that it wants—and craves—nutritious, wholesome foods.

The reason your brain can be rewired is largely related to its neuroplasticity, your brain's ability to change and adapt based on your experiences. The term "neuroplasticity" doesn't mean that the brain is like plastic. Rather, "neuro" describes neurons, the nerve cells that are the building blocks of the brain and nervous system, and "plasticity" refers to the brain's ability to be molded by experiences, or its malleability.

Neuroplasticity is at the heart of habit formation. By nature, your brain forms neuronal pathways based on what you do habitually. If you eat junk food a lot, for example, your neural pathways lead you to munching on chips while watching TV or eating dessert every night after dinner or grabbing a candy bar in midafternoon while working. Pretty soon, the bad habit becomes the unconscious default pathway, and your brain, wanting to be efficient, just takes the easiest, most familiar route. Along with all this repetitive behavior, your brain gets so used to processed foods that you start to crave them.

A lot of this habitual behavior has to do with dopamine, and I'll elaborate on that in a moment. Interestingly, habits are not created equally. Behaviors that churn out the most dopamine are the most habit-forming. This is one big way addictions are born. For example, smoking triggers a big hit of dopamine. It doesn't take many cigarettes to pick up the practice before you're hooked. Eating sugar also signals a dopamine burst. Compare these habits to, say, flossing your teeth, which doesn't provide any such dopamine surge.

Still, you can change your eating habits—and even balance dopamine releases—to curb your intake of sugar and junk food, and instead start habitually eating healthier foods like fruits and veggies. As you do this more often, you override those previous pesky neural pathways with new ones, liberating you from entrenched poor eating habits. Choosing healthy foods becomes a second-nature habit, and you do it automatically.

Until the completion of my fellowship and three years of clinical work, I had no idea that there was so much powerful science behind neuroplasticity. Once the light bulb went on, I was able to overhaul my habits and completely transform my health, my mind, and the way I lived. I was able to change my brain. And you will too.

With Step 2, you'll rewire your brain so that you naturally gravitate toward better, more satisfying food preferences. The process involves several easy strategies that you can implement right away. Keep reading to find out what I mean.

## INTERMITTENT REWARD SCHEDULING

Let's get back to our old friend dopamine. It's the brain chemical responsible for pleasure, motivation, drive, cravings, and movement.

In his Huberman Lab podcast *How to Increase Motivation, and Drive,* Dr. Andrew Huberman, who was introduced in Chapter 1, explains that your brain and body both have baseline levels of dopamine, the amount that is circulating all the time. Your baseline is important in regulating how you feel, whether you're in a good mood, feel motivated and driven, and find pleasure in various activities.

You also experience peaks in dopamine above your baseline. Different factors, good and bad, can stimulate these peaks. When you experience pleasure from activities like having sex, eating sugary foods, gambling, using drugs, or even intense physical exercise, dopamine can spike. These spikes light up the pleasure centers of the brain, sending signals saying that whatever is being done at that moment—running, eating, making love, and so forth—is pleasurable, encouraging us to do these things, and driving us to do them more often.

Our dopamine system, with its baseline and peaks, is an evolutionary holdover from the days of our hunter-gatherer ancestors. Eons ago, early humans needed to know what types of foods to forage for and which animals to hunt. All of these primal desires were driven by dopamine and enabled early humans to survive in the wild and pass down their genes. Basically, without dopamine in the brains of early humans, we wouldn't be here today. The dopamine system is a survival mechanism that has perpetuated the human species.

Dopamine, however, is also one of the reasons food becomes addictive. Sugar and fat are two substances that affect dopamine production in the brain; both can be addicting on their own and are especially potent when combined, as they are in processed foods. (Recall how we talked earlier about the ways in which the food industry engineers food to be addictive.) Other stimulants such as alcohol and drugs can also influence this neurotransmitter.

As your body produces more dopamine in response to an influx of sugar and fat—these are the peaks I'm talking about—dopamine starts to dip below the baseline. That's not good because the body needs to maintain this baseline for basic drive, motivation, and locomotion. When dopamine falls below the baseline, you then need to eat more and more junk food to feel the same way as when you started eating or to catch the same dopamine high. (Note that drug and alcohol addictions work in a similar way.) Essentially, the body develops a tolerance, addiction sets in, and you crave more sugar or fat—or both.

Now here's the kicker: you can break a food addiction by achieving healthy peaks in dopamine activity and by maintaining your baseline. The question is: How?

The key lies in a practice called intermittent reward scheduling. This happens to be the central way casinos keep you gambling (sometimes you hit the jackpot and sometimes you don't), an elusive or potential love interest keeps you on the hook, or social media sites motivate and engage you by offering you likes. All of these situations provide a dopamine hit.

These examples highlight the more negative applications of intermittent reward scheduling, but there are positive uses too. For example, you can employ it to halt cravings for junk food. Intermittent reward scheduling can actually rewire your brain so that you are not constantly craving sweets or junk food, or falling into addictive patterns with foods you crave.

This works because dopamine actually flows much more readily when the rewards, such as a piece of dark chocolate or a cookie, are intermittent and random—for example, you don't get to eat a cinnamon bun every time you see one. Instead, you eat one at intermittent but arbitrary times. Intermittent reward scheduling is very easy to incorporate into your life, and forms a key part of my 3-2-1 technique, which I'll explain next.

## PRACTICE MY 3-2-1 TECHNIQUE

This technique combines intermittent reward scheduling with certain strategies used in cognitive behavioral therapy (CBT), a form of psychological treatment that works effectively for a range of problems, including depression, anxiety, addictions, eating disorders, and severe mental illness, among others. Unlike many forms of therapy, CBT helps you change faulty or unhelpful ways of thinking. For example, you learn how to recognize distortions in thinking that are creating problems, then change thinking patterns so that they are more in line with reality.

Here's a specific example that relates to how you might view food: When you eat a candy bar, how do you normally feel afterward? Happy and content? Or guilty and ashamed?

A lot of people feel bad after eating a candy bar, or something they consider forbidden, and they get upset with themselves. The thought process goes something like: "I ate a bad food; therefore, I'm a bad person." This reaction is inaccurate and irrational—food is not a moral arbiter of your character. In other words, eating a so-called bad food doesn't make you a bad person, nor does eating a good food make you a good person.

CBT helps you make a psychological shift in your thinking regarding that particular food, so that eating it doesn't cause negative feelings. I read an intriguing study published in the journal *Appetite* in which participants were asked if they associated chocolate cake more with guilt or with celebration. Those who said they felt guilty after eating chocolate cake had more health issues and problems with motivation than those who associated the cake with celebration. In fact, the guilty eaters felt out of control around food and said they were more likely to overeat.

Here's the problem: Feelings of guilt and shame over food only trigger other negative feelings, like helplessness and lack of control, and increase self-criticism. All of these responses can snowball into poor self-esteem, a depressed or anxious mood, and further cravings. It's thus important to disassociate negative feelings from food in order to minimize cravings. CBT helps you do that. Next I'll explain how this works and show you how to practice my 3-2-1 technique. Make sure you read through the instructions entirely before starting the technique to understand how the three components overlap and are used together.

*The 3 component.* The first week, select three days—say, Monday, Wednesday, and Friday—on which to enjoy a chosen treat, such as two squares of dark chocolate or a couple of oatmeal cookies.

The next week do the same, but on three different days, such as Tuesday, Thursday, and Saturday.

Keep changing the schedule up each week, never following a predictable timeline. This unreliability provides dopamine peaks but without depleting your baseline. By adding the element of uncertainty to the same reward, you maintain a healthy balance of your dopamine levels. The higher the level of unpredictability of a reward, the more you maintain your baseline of dopamine, produce modest peaks, and stop ever-increasing cravings for sweets and junk food.

*The 2 component.* When you sit down to have a treat, first spend 2 minutes going through the following CBT exercise.

- Restructure your thoughts. Instead of saying "Ugh, I hate myself for eating this," say something nice to yourself—something you would say to a best friend who is struggling with sugar cravings. For example: "Good job, Allison, for picking a treat for yourself that is healthy and nutritious rather than the processed treats of your past. You are moving forward."

- Journal or mentally answer the following questions: What are you doing for self-care this week? Prioritizing sleep? Getting out in nature? Making nutritious food choices? Enjoying friends and family? The more you focus on the positive choices you're making, the more your triggers for cravings will dissipate.
- Let yourself relax prior to eating something that normally provokes guilt, shame, or anxiety. Release the tension in your head, jaw, shoulders—really your whole body—and see how recharged you feel. Then release any negative feelings about the food. Welcome it as a pure treat that you will enjoy without remorse. This attitude begins to rewire your brain to think differently about that food.

*The 1 component.* Sit your a\*\* down for one minute (I know I sound like a stern mother, but when it comes to neuroplasticity, you have to be strict with yourself!) and do the following.

- Once you're relaxed, eat the treat. Give yourself permission to savor it. Concentrate on the flavor, the aroma, and the texture. Continue to tune out any thoughts, especially about the moral value of the food.
- Register a mental note of what you enjoyed about eating the food—its taste, its crunch, its aroma, the surroundings in which you enjoyed it, and so forth. This practice forges a positive association with the food that can be reinforced in the future with repetition.

I worked with Tina to employ my 3-2-1 technique. I also suggested that she add the Super Six from Step 1 to her diet each day, to further help with her sugar addiction and begin to rewire her brain.

Guess what? Her sugar cravings markedly subsided within two weeks. By four weeks, as with most people who use this technique, Tina had conquered the addiction and felt completely liberated from the grip that sweets had held over her life.

Try the 3-2-1 technique. It will require your brain to think differently about food and curb your cravings substantially. You will learn to focus not so much on what you think you can't eat but rather on all the delicious dishes you can enjoy, and on the foods you can add to your diet rather than those you leave out. Then wave goodbye to cravings.

## Cravings Crusher: Dopamine and Caffeine

One way to balance dopamine—that is, maintain your baseline and modulate your peaks—is to drink caffeinated beverages like coffee, tea, or yerba mate in moderation (one to three cups daily, preferably prior to noon so that your caffeine consumption does not interfere with your sleep).

Caffeine does not spike dopamine like other stimulants (for example, nicotine, cocaine, or amphetamines) do. Rather, it has been shown to increase dopamine receptors on cells. For perspective, receptors are like locks, while the substances binding to them—in this case, dopamine—are the keys to those locks. The more dopamine receptors, the more dopamine there is to access cells and do its work. More research is needed in this area, but the fact that caffeine increases dopamine receptors suggests that it may help balance dopamine and thus possibly calm cravings.

Postscript: Coffee is a mild appetite suppressant. A constituent of coffee is a group of plant antioxidants called chlorogenic acids that can help curb hunger. Coffee also contains the hunger-suppressing hormone PYY (peptide tyrosine tyrosine). It is released into blood cells in the lining of the small intestine and colon, where it goes to work helping you feel full and satiated.

# ADJUST YOUR EATING BEHAVIOR
# A LITTLE AT A TIME

Honestly, we didn't come into this world loving French fries and hating, for example, a nice baked sweet potato. Over time we are conditioned to prefer—highly processed, ultrapalatable foods. This is a learned behavior that is reinforced in response to eating them—repeatedly. But as I explained in Chapter 4, any behavior that is learned can be unlearned. We can train our brains to desire healthy foods over less healthy foods.

In a pilot study published in the journal *Nutrition & Diabetes*, scientists demonstrated this very point—that altering your eating behavior can actually change how your brain reacts to various foods. They split thirteen overweight and obese participants into two groups: a control group and an experimental group. At the start of the study, both groups underwent brain scans to record their brain activity in response to photos of various foods.

The experimental group then participated in a behavioral intervention program. They followed portion-controlled menus that consisted of healthy, high-fiber, high-protein (nutrient-dense) foods and were designed to prevent hunger and cravings. They also participated in support group sessions. The control group simply continued their regular way of eating.

After six months, people in the experimental group had lost an average of 14 pounds, while the control group had lost about 5 pounds.

Both groups were rescanned, while researchers showed the participants photos of nutrient-dense foods, like a turkey sandwich, and high-calorie foods, such as French fries. They compared how the brains of the different groups of participants responded to these photos, particularly in an area known to be associated with the brain's reward system.

Remember that other studies mentioned in this book have shown that high-calorie, fatty, sugary foods trigger the reward centers of the brain. That's why you naturally crave these foods.

But in this experiment, the results of the second scans revealed that seeing photos of healthy food caused the brains of the people in the experimental group to light up! Researchers actually saw less activity in the brains of those participants when they were shown junky foods and more activity when they were shown nutrient-rich foods. The same results did not hold true for the control group.

In short, the experimental group was no longer craving foods like French fries, as shown by the brain scans. They desired the healthier choice!

Slowly introducing nutritious, satiating foods into your diet—like the Super Six nutrients listed in Step 1—is another way to rewire your brain so that you will gradually be less tempted by processed, junk, or fast foods. The meal plans in Chapter 10 will help you do this.

**Cravings Crusher:** Think About Junk Food Differently

Try this experiment from researchers at the University of Oregon, published in the journal *Appetite*, which helps people look at their favorite junk food in a negative light. The researchers asked participants to try one or more of the following strategies:

1. Imagine that you are feeling very full.

2. Focus on the bad outcomes of eating that food (such as a stomachache or weight gain).

3. Remind yourself that you can save that food for later.

4. Imagine that something bad has happened to the food (such as being sneezed on).

Guess what happened? These strategies lessened the participants' cravings and desire for junk food. Your mind is pretty powerful. Give this experiment a try and see what happens!

# THINK OF YOURSELF AS A
# HEALTHFUL EATER

Another simple strategy to rewire your brain is to think of yourself as a healthful eater. This mindset makes it easier to stick to healthy food choices. That's according to a U.S. study, published in the *Journal of Health Psychology*, which found that when people trying to implement a dietary change, such as eating more fruit, created a new label for themselves—like fruit eater—their eating behavior followed suit. The researchers say it's purely psychological: the more you identify with a particular role, like healthy eater, the more likely you are to start participating in role-related behaviors, including healthy eating, without trying too hard!

Also, stop saying "I can't eat sweets/fast food" and so forth. Instead, phrase your preference as "I don't" more often—much like vegans and vegetarians say "I don't eat meat." A study in the *Journal of Consumer Research* noted that when people used the words "I don't" to describe their trigger foods, they were less likely to choose crappy foods than people who said "I can't."

Why are such words important? Researchers believe that saying "I don't" is psychologically empowering. It implies that the decision is yours to make, and that you are in control.

As you truly become a healthful eater, start noticing the effects of foods you choose—right after you eat them and continuing into the next day. For example, how do you feel after a big meal of fried, fatty foods or overly sugary treats? Not so good, I bet.

Then compare those observations to how you feel after a day or two of eating clean, healthful foods with real nutritional value. Notice your energy levels, the quality of your sleep, and the clarity of your thinking, among other benefits. Focusing on these good feelings creates new pathways in your brain that associate health and happiness with eating whole, natural foods.

## Hunger Hack: Survive the Buffet Line

Almost daily, millions of restaurant patrons, conference attendees, college students, armed services personnel, and others, and maybe even you—serve themselves at buffets, many of the all-you-can-eat variety. But buffets can be a dangerous place. Although they may save your wallet from emptying, they can be a nightmare if you're trying to stay healthy and stabilize your weight. Here's the trick to surviving the pitfalls of a buffet when serving yourself a meal: start with a cup of broth-based soup or a salad. Either one will fill you up. From there, pile veggies on your plate. They are filling as well. Enjoy those, and you won't go overboard on unhealthy choices.

## TRY A DOPAMINE DETOX

Here's one more tool you can try when working to rewire your brain: a dopamine detox. This involves fasting from dopamine-producing activities for a period a of time, with the goal of breaking the pattern of addictive behaviors like mindlessly eating junk food and being hooked on sugary foods, as well as excessive alcohol drinking, doing recreational drugs, gambling, gaming, and so forth. Although there is no scientific evidence to support this method, you might want to try it if you're tired of emotional eating, dealing with lots of cravings, or just want to build a better relationship with food.

To clarify: Although the term "dopamine detox" may suggest otherwise, you can't get addicted to dopamine itself. When released, this neurotransmitter positively reinforces the behavior or activity that caused it to be released. That behavior or activity becomes associated with the dopamine release, leading to an addiction to it—not to dopamine.

To try a dopamine detox, I have several suggestions to help you. First, zero in on which behavior you want to detox. Eating too many sweets? Diving into a bag of chips at night while watching TV? Excessive alcohol consumption? You know what you need to unplug from!

- Make it difficult to engage in the behavior. Get rid of the offending substance or at least put it out of sight.
- Set a period of time in which you will not eat sugar, sweets, chips, or other junk food. It could be a week or multiple weeks.
- Engage yourself in activities to distract you from the behavior, such as reading, journaling, exercising, taking up a new hobby, and so forth.

Take note of how you feel after you have detoxed and hopefully decreased your dopamine-reward sensitivity. You might find that you have developed a healthier relationship with food, with your body, and with your life as a whole.

**Cravings Crusher:** Break a Bad Habit in One Easy Step

Habits, good or bad, have purpose: to free our brains up for more important challenges. In other words, they put us on autopilot so we can manage our lives more easily. Of course, there are habits that serve us well, like eating healthy foods, exercising, flossing, and so forth; other habits are harmful, such as smoking, eating junk food, or being sedentary.

It's those harmful habits we want to break, and there is an easy way to do it. Let's say you want to break your habit of munching on chips while you watch TV. If you can break that habit, you'll go a long way toward managing your hunger and cravings, since eating junk food only worsens hunger signals.

The key is to pair that bad habit with a good habit immediately afterward. Start by bringing conscious awareness to the bad habit—the one you want to break. Then engage in a positive replacement behavior immediately. For example, after eating those chips, do something that you deem positive—maybe it's drinking a glass of water or eating an apple, doing some deep breathing or meditating, taking a walk in nature, or the like. Following a bad habit with a good one overrides your neural circuits. The bad habit will ease its grip on you, and you'll begin to build positive habits that will help you achieve your health goals.

So, to end cravings and food addiction, there's hope and lots of it. Rewiring your brain to avoid cravings and stop food addiction is a matter of understanding how your body works, including how your brain thinks about food, and then changing its pathways. Practice these techniques, fuel your body with the Super Six nutrients in Step 1, and you'll find that you can make it through the day without craving foods that interfere with your health. Once you start selecting foods with real nutritional value, you will actually get hooked on them!

# 7

## Step 3: Reset

IN THE FALL OF 2021, which was the first time I could really travel outside the U.S. in over a year due to the pandemic, I took a vacation to Spain with my good friend, Priti. We spent five days in Majorca and Madrid, enjoying the European culture and food.

During the vacation, I stopped my usual healthy habits such as eating vegetables and avoiding refined carbohydrates. I also did not stick to my early dinner schedule, because people in Spain don't eat dinner until nine or ten o'clock at night. I stepped right into the local culture, and I did have fun. However, my digestion was definitely affected—and not in a good way!

After an amazing vacation, I flew home to my normal time zone. Once home, I experienced a strange phenomenon. The first week I was back, I'd wake up ravenously hungry—as if it was time for dinner. I would then eat an early, full meal of beans, vegetables, and rice—similar to the dinners I had while in Spain.

At home, I don't eat breakfast that early, and I don't eat a huge meal for breakfast. Something was off!

I normally break my fast after my workout. You may have read in my first book, *I'm So Effing Tired,* that I practice something called circadian fasting (see page 114 of this book for more information): I avoid food for a certain period of time, work out, then eat my first meal at 10 A.M., after my workout.

My vacation caused my hunger signals to become completely effed up! This experience illustrated to me that hunger often comes in circadian patterns.

Normally, we feel tired at night and get hungry around specific times of the day. That's because our bodies have a built-in process that governs sleep, hunger, and energy levels. It's called circadian rhythm, from the Latin words *circa,* meaning "around," and *dies,* meaning "day." The circadian rhythm repeats roughly every twenty-four hours to maximize our body's own resources. We share this rhythm with all life on earth, from plants to animals, and even bacteria.

The circadian rhythm is our own internal clock that regulates the sleep–wake cycle, manages hunger, influences brain-wave activity patterns, affects cell repair, controls body temperature, impacts hormone release, and is involved in our eating habits and digestion. However, if you're like most people, you'll notice the effect of circadian rhythm on your sleep patterns. Since writing *I'm So Effing Tired,* I've gotten hundreds of questions about circadian rhythm, especially how it affects hunger.

For thousands of years before electricity was invented, humans awoke with the sun and went to bed when it was dark. It was a lovely natural rhythm we shared with nature, and a natural rhythm we still carry with us today in many ways, as our internal clocks are set by this pattern.

My first experience with circadian rhythm occurred years ago— when I did my residency at Harvard Medical School's Beth Israel Deaconess Medical Center in Boston. I was a little burned out from medical school and had just gotten married, so my start there was brutal. The hours were worse than in med school, and I found myself unusually tired and hungry throughout the long workdays. Boston just happens to get dark very early many months out of the year. I'd go to work at 6 A.M., and it would be pitch black. When I left work in the evening, guess what, it would still be pitch black. *Get me out of here!* I thought. That's when I found out the hard way how our circadian rhythm was altering my hunger, cravings, mood, and energy during Boston's dark winters.

In recent years, we've learned a lot about circadian rhythm and what it means for our health. For instance, we've known for a long time that we have an inner clock composed of a group of neurons called the suprachiasmatic nucleus (which sounds awfully like the song "Supercalifragilisticexpialidocious" in *Mary Poppins*) that resides in the hypothalamus and affects our sleep–wake cycle. But what we didn't realize until recently—and we are only starting to understand—is that there are individual clocks in every cell in every one of our organs, and they can function even without the central circadian clock.

Every cell has this inner clock, independent of the main one in our brain. Just think about all the mini timers in our skin, muscles, digestive tract, heart, liver—all working on a set time. We also know that all our cells' mitochondria—the microscopic energy factors in cells—have a relationship with our circadian rhythm, and this affects the importance of when we eat, as well as what we eat.

Disturbances to the circadian rhythm, or to the genes that produce the rhythm, can abuse this beautiful timing by constantly changing our sleep patterns and eating schedules and exposing ourselves to unfriendly environments that mess with those inner clocks. Some of these disruptors include:

- Shift work with erratic hours that don't align with the natural light and dark times of day
- Unlimited access to and choice of different palatable, high-caloric foods and beverages
- Irregular eating patterns
- Travel that spans the course of one or more time zones, causing jet lag

- A lifestyle that encourages late-night hours or early wake times
- Stressful situations in life
- Poor sleep habits, including an inconsistent sleep schedule, eating, or drinking late at night, watching TV or looking at computer screens too close to bedtime, or not having a comfortable sleeping space (more on all this in the next chapter!)

Clearly, most of these alterations of circadian biology are caused by modern life, and they have a bad influence on our cells and our hormone production, including that of our hunger hormones. In fact, our hunger hormones do not like these disruptions!

Scientists have learned a great deal about circadian rhythms by studying organisms with similar biological clock genes, such as fruit flies and mice. In 2017, Jeffrey C. Hall, Michael Rosbash, and Michael W. Young won the Nobel Prize in Physiology or Medicine for discovering the molecular mechanisms that underpin these extremely important biological clocks. In experiments with fruit flies, which have genes that correspond to those in humans, they isolated a gene that helps govern circadian rhythm. This gene manufactures a protein that accumulates in cells overnight, then degrades during the day. All of this impacts when you sleep, how well your brain works, and more.

Other exciting findings have been discovered since then and shed further light on how circadian rhythm regulates hunger. For example, when genes that control circadian rhythm are deleted, mice tend to become obese and process glucose differently, suggesting that hunger/satiety responses in animals are governed by circadian rhythm. Likewise, turning off clock genes in mouse AgRP neurons, which are central command for hunger and satiety, disrupts the animals' feeding patterns. Normally, mice (which are nocturnal) consume about 80 percent of their food at night. But the mice whose clock genes were turned off ate more food during the day, when they'd usually be sleeping.

So—circadian rhythm and hunger? Yes, they're controlled all the way down at the genetic level of our bodies.

For managing hunger and cravings, resetting your natural circadian rhythm is paramount—and it's what Step 3 is all about.

---

## Is Your Circadian Rhythm Out of Whack?

If so, you'll feel it. Here are some telltale signs:

- Extreme hunger and cravings at odd times
- Difficulty falling asleep or staying asleep
- Daytime sleepiness or sleepiness during shift work
- Fatigue or exhaustion
- Poor concentration
- Less alertness
- Poor control over emotions and mood
- Headaches
- Digestive upset

---

## HOW TO RESET YOUR CIRCADIAN RHYTHM

Yes, it might sound scary to think about how modern life can mess with our circadian rhythm and make us ravenously hungry. But let me put you at ease. By following this step of my plan, you can make several simple changes that will help you recalibrate your system.

### Expose Yourself to Morning Light

Our circadian clocks get direct input from the sun. One of the best ways to help reset your circadian cycle is to expose yourself to the morning sunlight within an hour of waking. This helps stimulate regular cortisol production to provide you with energy for the day.

While cortisol is best known as the stress hormone, it also manages a host of other functions, including the task of waking

---

you up and getting you moving. Cortisol decreases throughout the morning and early afternoon, then jumps up a little again in mid-afternoon before declining again in preparation for sleep. Exposure to morning light helps set the stage for our sleep–wake cycle and regulates sleep patterns.

Try to expose yourself to as much natural light as you can throughout the day. Take a walk outside for lunch or sit by a window that lets in sunlight. Exposing yourself to daylight helps your body wake up and stay alert.

## Try Bright Light Therapy

This technique is a great way to reset your circadian rhythm. You can purchase a device, usually a lightbox or a lamp, on your own, but you may want to talk to a sleep professional about the level of exposure, what time of day, and how often and for how long you should expose yourself to these lights. Bright light therapy may be an excellent option for those who work late at night or early in the morning.

Additionally, bright light therapy may be helpful for those with seasonal affective disorder, a form of depression that can set in during winter months when exposure to natural light is limited.

## Fast to Reset Your Internal Clock

Because digestion and metabolism can play a role in your level of sleepiness and wakefulness, you may need to adjust when you eat and what you eat. Typically, animals adapt their circadian rhythms to match the availability of food. And some research has shown that you can fast for up to sixteen hours to help reset your internal clock. If you fast in this manner, it's essential to stick to regular mealtimes because once your body expects food at a specific time, eating then helps promote circadian rhythm.

My version of fasting is called circadian fasting. Following this method, you avoid food between the hours of 8 P.M. to 8 A.M., or 7 P.M. to 7 A.M.—a twelve-hour fasting period. You can also experience great benefits from a fourteen-hour fast, in which case your fasting window would be from 8 P.M. to 10 A.M. These fasting lengths may be less trendy than the longer sixteen-hour fast, but if we're going to reset our circadian clock, a twelve- or fourteen-hour fast is much more flexible, attainable, and manageable. Once you're comfortable with, say, a twelve-hour fast, you can work up to fasting sixteen hours two to three times a week, from 8 P.M. to noon the next day.

## Some Additional Fasting Guidelines

- Cluster most of your meals from 12 P.M. to 5 P.M. Try not to eat within three hours of bedtime, and do not overeat during your feeding window.
- Plan your meals and eating times in advance. A guide I follow is to break your fast with something small between 8 A.M. and 10 A.M., eat lunch at noon, and have dinner between 3 P.M. and 6 P.M. if your schedule allows.
- Make sure to include foods from the Super Six nutrients in Step 1 in your meals. My meal plans (see Chapter 10) will help you.
- If you get hungry during your fasting period, try to curb your hunger with some of my hunger hacks and cravings crushers. Also, have water or noncaloric drinks (such as coffee and tea). If your hunger does not dissipate, eat something that is sugar-free and is 40 calories or less, such as a spoonful of peanut butter, a thin slice of avocado, or a handful of nuts. (Fasting normally keeps hunger hormones in check, so you may not feel hungry at all.)
- Stay hydrated while fasting. Drink 80 to 100 ounces of water daily.
- Check that you are on the right path by asking yourself some questions and paying attention to what the answers tell you about your body: How's your sleep? How are your hunger and cravings? How's your energy? Are your monthly cycles still regular? Are you feeling better than you have in the past?

Monitoring yourself is a good way to gauge how well you are resetting your circadian rhythm.

- Get plenty of rest. Work on sleep hygiene for good quality sleep each night. Also, a twenty-minute nap during the day can do wonders for your body. If you can squeeze in a quick nap, take advantage of the chance to recharge. (Step 4, in Chapter 8, is all about refreshing through sleep and rest.)

---

### Hunger Hack: Stop Effing Hunger Throughout the Day

One way to feel less hungry all day is to push back your ghrelin secretion by about forty-five minutes to an hour in the morning. Let's say you usually prefer to eat your first meal at 7:30 A.M. In this case you will start the practice of circadian fasting by going twelve to sixteen hours without food following your dinner and your first meal. Much of this time will pass overnight while you're sleeping. Spend four or five days shifting your first meal, which was ordinarily breakfast at 7:30, so that you eat forty-five minutes to an hour later. By then, you'll be eating your first meal almost at 10:00 A.M. and you'll have trained your body not to secrete ghrelin during the morning hours.

You might assume that when your stomach is empty from fasting like this, more ghrelin would be released, making you ravenous. Surprisingly, this doesn't happen. Fasting actually turns off ghrelin and makes you less hungry.

Research provides proof. A study in the journal *Obesity* looked at the intermittent fasting method and found that after four days of fasting for sixteen hours and eating only within a six-hour window, those fasting had lower ghrelin levels overall than they did previously and said their hunger level was minimal.

---

# Eat at Regular Times

Do you ever postpone lunch because you're racing to meet a deadline? Or do you skip dinner when you work late? Nothing to worry about, right?

Well, maybe it is.

Research reported in the *Proceedings of the Nutrition Society* suggested that eating your meals on a hit-and-miss schedule may set you up for obesity, high blood pressure, type 2 diabetes, and problems with cholesterol and insulin levels. On a brighter note, the research found that adults who ate regular meals—at similar times from one day to the next—were less obese than people who ate their meals at irregular times.

It's pretty amazing, even a bit unusual, that the timing of your meals to match a set schedule could impact your health that much. Yet it does—and represents a fairly simply change you can make in meal planning and in your lifestyle. The whole interrelationship of nutrition, metabolism, and circadian rhythm is referred to as chrononutrition.

Chrononutrition, if you think about it, makes sense, considering that key metabolic processes in the body—such as appetite, digestion, and the metabolism in general—follow patterns that repeat every twenty-four hours. So eating meals at inconsistent or irregular times may mess up your internal body clock. And that disruption could lead to weight gain and other health risks.

Having irregular mealtimes rather than eating on a set schedule throws your body into stress mode, too. For example, if you have breakfast at 6 A.M. one day and 10 A.M. the next, your body will be confused about when its next meal is coming. Greater levels of the stress hormone cortisol are secreted. Soaring cortisol can then spike insulin, which causes inflammation and can increase the risk of disease.

It's clearly important to eat in sync with your circadian rhythm in order to manage hunger and improve your health. If you eat out of sync of this rhythm, you may be at a greater risk for cardiovascular disease, diabetes, and obesity.

So based on what we know, it's a good idea to eat at the same times every day if you can. I know doing so might be difficult, especially if you have a hectic schedule like mine—but do your best to establish some regularity in your eating patterns.

For more information on meal timing, go to my Resource Link at www.amymdwellness.com/timing for a graphic on how to plan your meals and your day to naturally manage your hunger.

## Eat an Early Dinner

Because your circadian rhythm is also related to your eating habits, eating a late dinner can delay your sleep. That said, eat your last meal between two or three hours before you go to bed. This will give your body enough time to digest your food, and it can help you fall asleep. However, what you eat matters too—avoid heavy and high-fat meals right before you go to bed.

This recommendation optimizes your blood sugar and insulin, contributing not only to restful sleep but better overall health. Eating too close to bedtime, late at night, or in the middle of the night desynchronizes your internal clock, which leads to sleeplessness, cravings, and weight gain.

## Get Close to Nature

It's a no-brainer that getting out in nature and breathing in fresh air and experiencing quiet is good for the soul. There's something about being away from all the stimulation of an urban or suburban existence and wrapping yourself in natural scenery that creates a sense of calm and relaxes the nervous system.

Let's say you're camping, and the sun goes down. Your body senses changes in the light and temperature, both of which signal that it is time to sleep. In the morning, you wake up to natural sunlight (no alarm clock!), which tells your body that it is time to get up.

Spending more time in nature can help with circadian disruptions and set you on a path to start living the way the body was designed to live.

# Limit Your Stress Levels

Until recently, it was relatively unclear why stress has such a heavy influence on disease and health, but now we know that our circadian clocks and our stress response systems are closely related, and cortisol is one of the big aggravators here. If you are chronically stressed, cortisol is churned out in higher amounts throughout the day. This creates a cortisol imbalance—which, among other problems, makes sleeping difficult, a result of disturbing your circadian clock.

Cortisol constantly triggers circadian genes in your liver and adrenal cells. The net effect is that your body becomes disoriented and cannot sense what time it is. This can lead to circadian dys-regulation, in which your body does not secrete hormones at the right times as part of its normal process of supporting your normal sleep–wake cycle. What's more, this interference with your circadian rhythm leaves you feeling hungry and exhausted all the time.

Stress, then, is one of the great disruptors of circadian rhythm. I can relate, because cortisol was my personal nemesis—I experienced limited sleep, too much coffee, cravings, stress at work and at home. All of this threw me into a crisis. For me, getting my stress under control with sleep, meditation, and yoga was the biggest step I took to reset my own circadian rhythm.

How about you? Can I see a show of hands if you feel that your life is too stressful? Ah, that's just about everyone!

You're definitely not alone. The American Psychological Association reports that we are dealing with more stress than ever before and suffering extreme physical and emotional harm as a result.

If you want to reduce stress in your life, there are several ways I recommend:

- Practice yoga
- Meditate
- Listen to soothing music
- Take relaxing baths
- Eat foods rich in antioxidants such as fruits and vegetables
- Take deep, cleansing breaths

To these tips, I propose two others. One is to ground yourself in nature. There are around twenty studies so far suggesting that direct contact with the earth—being barefoot in the grass or on the beach—affects white blood cells, anti-inflammatory cellular proteins, and other molecules that regulate inflammation. This grounding in nature can help improve sleep, regulate cortisol, and alleviate stress. The feeling of the earth under your feet is not only soothing, but you may be absorbing electrons from the earth through your feet that help reduce inflammation and balance cortisol.

Also, I believe that it is important to work on changing your response to the stressors in your life. Here's the deal: it's not the problem (the stressor) itself that is stressing you out. Rather, it's your perception of the problem that is causing you stress. The Greek philosopher Epictetus made this point more than two thousand years ago: "People are disturbed not by events but by their view of them."

Therefore, the solution is to reframe your response to the stressor so that your stress level goes down. Yes, reframing your problem is easier said than done, especially when you're the one dealing with the stressor. I get it!

Try to keep in mind, though, that the stressor itself is neither positive nor negative. It is simply a neutral event in your life that has popped up. Your reaction to it is what creates stress.

What's the solution? Try to not let the stressor derail you. Change your reaction to it. For example, take a positive attitude and start viewing problems as challenges. Your self-talk will then change. Once that internal shift occurs, you'll move closer to constructively dealing with your stressor. Additionally, you will feel empowered rather than victimized. As a result, your quality of life will improve, and your stress level will decrease.

For example, I had a patient, Mariana, who is an infectious disease physician. Over the pandemic, she came to me in the poorest of health and mindset and downtrodden over the long, stressful days of treating covid-19 patients. She kept saying to me, "Why is this happening to me?" It was a question that was not helpful for reducing her stress level.

I asked her to reframe the issue by asking different questions: "What am I learning from this experience?" "How will I be a better doctor, mom, and person after coming out of this situation?"

I also asked her to focus on being thankful and grateful—a practice that trains the brain to see the good in your life. Together, with the other strategies here, Mariana started to improve her self-talk and ultimately her well-being. Positive self-talk is a big secret for reducing stress.

So take steps like these. These actions will not only make you feel calmer but allow you to avoid stress eating as a way of coping with your stressors. Modern life is filled with stressors, so finding ways to tone down their effects will help you feel and live more productively.

I wish I could tell you that there's a magic number that guarantees when your internal clock will completely reset, but it's a process that varies by individual. The length of time it will take to fix your circadian rhythm will depend on what is setting it off in the first place. Sometimes it might be jet lag from traveling, for example. After I got back from Spain, it took me a whole week to reset. But in other situations, it might take up to two weeks to adjust. Just know that by following Step 3—Reset—and its tips, you can go a long way toward keeping your biological clock in healthy sync.

# 8

## Step 4: Refresh

RIGHT AFTER SHE TURNED 45, Sara began to feel different. She couldn't quite put her finger on it, but things were definitely off.

"My sleep patterns now resemble a newborn's, and I'm not talking about 'sleeping like a baby.' I'm up every two hours. I toss and turn for hours every night, hoping my mind will shut off and let me go to sleep, but nope. I'm hungry all the time, too, and want to eat constantly."

To Sara, it seemed like her body was changing in other scary ways too. She was bloated and felt heavy and achy a lot of the time. It seemed like she had turned into Attila the Hun, snapping at everyone for no reason.

Sara told me she thought she had become possessed by a monster. I say this with my tongue in my cheek: the truth was worse. She was in perimenopause.

Perimenopause is the transitional time in a woman's life leading up to menopause. During perimenopause, which can last several years (yikes), hormones fluctuate considerably. It's a phase that has been likened to puberty in reverse, which means that it's like riding the scariest roller coaster you can imagine, except you're going backward.

Sara was not enjoying the transition, to say the least, especially the sleepless nights that left her exhausted the next day. Giving into the unrelenting hunger was no fun either. She was morphing into a heavier version of her normally fit self.

There is a happy ending to Sara's story—which I will get to later in this chapter.

Like Sara, have you ever felt ravenous or had uncontrollable urges for certain foods after tossing and turning? It's not just your imagination—and you don't even have to be in perimenopause or other states of hormonal flux—there's a proven link between poor quality sleep and hunger.

For instance, an article published in the journal *Nature* revealed that getting inadequate sleep for just one night may significantly increase your appetite, chances of overeating, and cravings for unhealthy food. Imagine that—just one night!

We've already talked a lot about the problem with sweets. Well, there is also evidence that eating more sugar can give you restless, disrupted sleep. In a 2016 study published in the *Journal of Clinical Sleep Medicine,* one group of volunteers followed a controlled diet that limited added sugars and fats and emphasized high-fiber foods. A second group was permitted to eat anything they wanted, in unlimited amounts.

The second group ate significantly more sugar and fat—and this had an impact on the quality of their nightly rest. They got very little deep, slow-wave sleep, which is essential for the body's nightly repair and healing, as well as for maintaining a healthy metabolism and immunity. The volunteers who ate more sugar also took longer to fall asleep. And they experienced more frequent awakenings throughout the night.

Here's something else: Your ability to think, reason, react, and respond slows with sleep deprivation. Researchers actually likened sleep deprivation to being intoxicated on alcohol. Plus, sleep affects the prefrontal cortex—that's the part of the brain that processes inhibition. So you'll be more likely to pick up things like junk food, cigarettes, or other addictive substances.

There's good news here, however. Researchers from the University of Cape Town in South Africa analyzed seven studies that focused on sleep duration. They found that when people got more sleep, they were less hungry during the day—and had fewer cravings for sweets and for salty foods. Their analysis was published in the journal *Nature*.

So—what does all this tell us? Sleep is a wonderful, natural appetite suppressant! Log in your *z*'s and sleep well, and you'll effortlessly get your hunger and cravings in check. This is what Step 4—Refresh—is all about.

## Sleepy Americans

We spend one-third of our lives asleep. Yet according to the Centers for Disease Control and Prevention, one out of every three Americans doesn't get enough sleep, likely because of work stress, family responsibilities, and daily house chores.

All adult human beings need at least seven to eight hours of sleep most nights. But why? Whether or not you feel the effects now, prolonged lack of sleep:

- Decreases brain power
- Weakens your immune response
- Kills your sex drive
- Increases cravings for carbohydrates and sugar
- Ages your skin
- Depletes your energy
- Puts you at risk for heart disease, diabetes, and some cancers
- Screws with your hormones

> If you continue to get less than the right amount of sleep, you might literally be taking years off your life by denying your body and mind the sleep it needs. A study from researchers in the United Kingdom who published in the journal *Sleep* found that people who went from seven hours to five hours or less of sleep a night suffered a 1.7-fold increased risk of premature death from all causes.
>
> Getting seven hours of sleep a night might just save your life!

## IT'S ALL ABOUT HORMONES—AGAIN!

So what exactly is going on? Why is the link between sleep issues and hunger so strong?

In a word: hormones.

Sleep deprivation as well as poor-quality sleep messes with levels of key hormones, so you feel hungry throughout the day. Several hormones are affected by sleep—which in turn make us hungrier than normal.

Let's look at the pivotal hormones that are involved in sleep and hunger, especially when it comes to sleep quality and sleep deprivation. While many hormones become off-kilter from poor sleep, we'll concentrate on the ones that make you ravenous when they're unbalanced and leave you yearning for a box of glazed doughnuts or huge slice of chocolate cake. Unbalanced ghrelin and leptin are the two most common culprits here, but insulin, cortisol, and melatonin have roles to play, too.

### Ghrelin and Leptin

Sleep plays an integral role in regulating the hormones leptin and ghrelin, which govern hunger and appetite. Ghrelin triggers hunger, and leptin triggers satiety. While you are in dreamland, your brain and your immune system are being restored and fortified, plus regulating ghrelin and leptin. If you don't get enough quality sleep, levels of this hormone rise, and with them comes an increased appetite. Leptin falls too, compounding hunger issues.

Research has found that ghrelin levels can shoot up 15 percent higher in people who sleep only five hours at night versus eight hours. So you know how you tend to get hungry when you're tired? Now you know why that happens!

## Growth Hormone (GH)

GH is responsible for your physical development. It can make you tall and muscular like your aunt Betty or petite like your aunt Sue. It's released at night, and you get another little burst in the early morning. GH repairs the skin, gut, and muscles. It also promotes cognitive function and overall well-being.

Important for the nightly secretion of GH is deep, non-REM (rapid eye movement) sleep, which occurs early in the night and predominates during the first third of the night. The less hours of sleep you log, the less of this wonder hormone your body will release. And, if you stay up all night or sleep at off hours, GH is not released at all. It's also important to know that if you toss and turn at night, then resume normal sleep, the brain releases extra GH; however, this throws off the natural balance of this hormone, and over time, less GH is secreted.

## Insulin

Another hormone affected by sleep is insulin. This hormone allows your body to use glucose from carbohydrates for energy or to store them for the future. Too little sleep may cause insulin resistance, in which the body can't use insulin properly, leading to blood sugar spikes and the possibility of diabetes and obesity.

Between 4 and 8 A.M., your body experiences a surge in glucose. If insulin does its job properly (no insulin resistance), it takes care of this situation and ushers glucose into cells for fuel. Your body uses the least glucose during REM (rapid eye movement) sleep and the most when you're awake.

A growing body of studies has shown that shortchanging sleep, even for only one night, disrupts insulin and glucose levels by creating insulin resistance, which can cause serious health issues including diabetes, cardiovascular disease, heart attacks, strokes, and even cancer.

In one trial, published in the *Journal of Diabetes Investigation*, more than four thousand people recorded how much sleep they got each night. Those who logged in less than six hours were twice as likely to have cells that were resistant to insulin or they had full-blown diabetes. This tells us that getting a good night's sleep on a regular basis helps your body use insulin efficiently—and can possibly help prevent type 2 diabetes and other insulin-related health problems. By the same token, having type 2 diabetes or insulin resistance is known to cause sleep disturbances.

But, according to the National Sleep Foundation, you can reverse any negative effects of sleep deprivation with a just couple nights of proper, uninterrupted sleep. (My sleep strategies later in this chapter will help you do this.)

## Cortisol

Cortisol is one of the main stress hormones, but as I've mentioned, it also manages a host of other functions, like helping the body better utilize carbohydrates, fats, and proteins; decreasing inflammation; stabilizing blood pressure; and normalizing your sleep–wake cycle.

From Step 3, you learned that the sleep–wake cycle follows a circadian rhythm. Every twenty-four hours, roughly synchronized with nighttime and daytime, your body enters a period of sleep followed by a waking period. The production of cortisol in your body follows a similar circadian rhythm.

Cortisol production drops to its lowest point around midnight and peaks about an hour after you wake up. For many people, the peak happens around 9 A.M., which is good timing because it makes us alert for the day.

In addition to the circadian cycle, around fifteen to eighteen smaller pulses of cortisol are released throughout the day and night. Some of those bursts correspond to shifts in your sleep cycles.

When you can't sleep or do not sleep well, your body will secrete more cortisol at night, further interrupting your sleep.

## Melatonin

Melatonin is the sleep hormone. It's manufactured by the pineal gland, located in the middle of the brain, and is released only at night. This hormone helps regulate the body's circadian rhythm. Darkness triggers its secretion but light, whether natural or artificial, blocks melatonin secretion.

It has many other functions too, like helping the body recover from exercise, acting as an antioxidant to strengthen the immune system, synchronizing your sleep–wake cycles, regulating blood pressure, and supporting the female reproductive cycle.

Melatonin does not affect hunger or appetite, per se, but it influences the action of ghrelin, leptin, and insulin—all of which orchestrate appetite, satiety, calorie uptake, and fat storage.

---

### Hunger Hack: Overeating and Sleep

Many clients have told me that since following my 5-step plan, plus rebooting their diets, they no longer overeat and they find it easier to fall asleep. Plus, they wake up less often during the night, and they rise in the morning feeling better rested and more energized. I'm thrilled about all of these results, of course, but I'm not totally surprised.

One huge benefit of the 5-step plan is that you stop habitual overeating, naturally and without the use of willpower. This benefit is supremely important. Overeating can mess up normal sleep. After a big dinner, for example, your body must devote energy to digestion, which typically takes several hours. But digestion normally slows down

---

during sleep. That hefty dinner pits your normal sleep process against the stomach's needs for digestion. A couple of very unpleasant symptoms can arise—like a tummy ache or, worse, painful acid reflux.

Large meals can also interfere with your sleep by raising the temperature of your body—which is the opposite to the body's typical process of cooling down during sleep. All of these problems make it very difficult to sleep through the night or get much-needed quality sleep.

If you're struggling with sleep issues, perhaps this information can help motivate you to get serious about improving your sleep habits!

## Assess Your Sleep

How's your sleep quality? Here's an assessment to help you find out. Take it now, then after a month of practicing my sleep skills, retake it to gauge any improvements in your sleep.

To test: Read the following statements and answer yes or no to each.

1. It takes me 30 or more minutes to fall asleep at bedtime.
   Yes or No

2. I rarely remember my dreams.
   Yes or No

3. I wake up in the morning still feeling tired and not very rested.
   Yes or No

4. I feel hungry more often, especially for junk food.
   Yes or No

5. I wake up earlier in the morning than I would like to.
   Yes or No

6. I sometimes feel sleepy and tired throughout the day.
   Yes or No

7. I frequently wake up one or more times during the night.
   Yes or No

8. I often lie awake at night and my mind races with worry
   and other thoughts.
   Yes or No

9. My eyes are puffy or red, or I have dark circles or bags
   under them in the morning.
   Yes or No

10. My emotions are all over the map—anger, impulsivity,
    anxiety, sadness, and so forth.
    Yes or No

To score: If you answered yes to three or more of these
statements, then likely you aren't getting enough sleep
or good-quality sleep. Start practicing the suggestions in
this step.

## TIME TO REFRESH!

Step 4 provides a set of practices collectively designed to help you
refresh so that your sleep-related hormones become balanced, your
body clock normalizes, and your hunger urges and cravings become
a thing of the past.

Now for Sara's happy ending. These are the exact sleep hygiene
practices I put her on. As a result, she got control of her sleep first
and then her hunger and cravings. She supported these actions with
natural hormone-balancing strategies that included greater intake of
omega-3 fatty acids, beans and legumes, and fresh fruits and vegetables. Great nutrition is always a wonderful natural treatment to correct
hormonal havoc and have the most immediate effect. Here is what's
involved.

## Change Your Mindset

When I was writing my first book, *I'm So Effing Tired*, I was not sleeping well, mostly due to stressing out over the deadline, taking care of my family, and dealing with hormonal issues related to my period. (Ironic given the topic of the book, I know.) On top of all that, I was stressed out about not getting a good night's sleep!

Yes, the Centers for Disease Control and Prevention recommends that adults need more than seven hours of sleep each night. But my life is busy, so is yours, and getting that much sleep isn't always in the cards.

I love to exercise in the morning but I also understand the importance of sleep—so I dug into my own lousy sleep schedule. Well, I discovered that if you're in a situation in which you have to choose between getting a little sleep or getting a workout in, it's better to opt for some sleep. But it's also not worth stressing if you can't get a full seven hours every night.

Ideally, aim for at least two good nights of sleep when life is busy—seven to eight hours each week, in other words. Sleeping well for two nights like this gives your body time to complete one full sleep cycle. Not only that, but you won't be so groggy when you wake up. In fact, you'll even feel refreshed the next day. This strategy was a real game changer for me. I was relieved that I didn't need to aim for a perfect sleep schedule of seven or more hours every single night.

## Sleep in the Dark and Get Lots of Light in the Morning

Circadian rhythm is controlled by the area of the brain that responds to light. So, in order to help support your natural secretions of melatonin, make sure to always sleep in the dark, and get lots of light in the daytime. Hang blackout shades in your bedroom and expose yourself to sunlight in the morning—for example, exercise, work, and walk outside if you can.

Beware of blue light from electronic screens such as your computer, smartphone, and similar devices. Blue light can confuse our body into delaying the production of melatonin. Therefore, if we look at screens until bedtime, the chances are high that we won't be able to fall asleep. I wear blue light-blocking glasses for computer or phone work in the evenings.

## Synchronize Your Circadian Rhythm

Go to bed and wake up at the same time every day, including weekends. Although, the exact times may vary, I am generally in bed between 9 P.M. and 10 P.M. and wake up between 5:30 A.M. and 7 A.M. Even on weekends I naturally wake up each morning at the same time. If you synchronize your sleeping and waking schedules like this, you will too.

For those fun nights out, I'll still wake up at my usual time and then fit in a quick nap (twenty minutes) later in the day so I'll have extra energy for going out.

## Cut Back on Cortisol-Triggering Foods

Yes, certain foods throw your cortisol out of balance—which means it can get high at night when it needs to be low so you can sleep well. Try to limit animal proteins, refined sugars, salt, and saturated fat. They all stimulate an over-release of cortisol. Diets rich in fruits and vegetables, on the other hand, are thought to promote the healthy cortisol production rhythms needed for sound, regular sleep.

## Avoid Sleep Wreckers

These include caffeine (in excess), alcohol, and nicotine. Caffeine in excess is a stimulant. Recent findings suggest that an evening cup of coffee alters circadian rhythms at the cellular level—so try to avoid it after noon. Try a glass of warm milk or decaffeinated tea if you need a beverage before bedtime.

Because it's a sedative, alcohol can make you sleepy at first but ultimately leads to disrupted sleep as liver enzymes metabolize it. The resulting poor sleep can also lead to excessive daytime sleepiness the following day.

Nicotine is also a stimulant. Smoking or vaping within four hours of bedtime disrupts your sleep quality and causes you to awaken frequently at night. Daily smokers suffer a lot of daytime sleepiness. In fact, research shows that people who smoke often (have their first puff early in the day) sleep for a shorter amount of time, with irregular sleep patterns.

Synthetic (and even natural) sleep aids and medications might help in the short term but ultimately will lead to an inability to fall asleep naturally over time.

## Don't Hang Out in Bed

To the best of your ability, make your bed and bedroom for sleeping and sex only. All other activities should be done somewhere else so that you unconsciously associate your bed with sleeping. If you watch TV, work, shop online, or eat in bed—and have trouble sleeping, keep those activities out of your bed and bedroom.

## Keep It Cool

Your bedroom, that is. Cool temperatures of 60 to 68 degrees Fahrenheit are close to our own internal body temperature (which drops to its lowest level when we sleep) and are the best temperatures for sleeping. Temperatures above or below this range seem to breed restless sleep.

Taking a cold shower can help cool down the body before bed.

## Destress to Rest

If your sleep is restless or you wake up at 3 A.M. and can't fall back to sleep, it's likely because your mind is racing—that is, you are experiencing anxiety or mental stress.

Listening to meditation or relaxation guides or sounds can be helpful. Do what you can to not bring things that cause you stress to bed with you. Don't go to bed angry, either, or engage in stress-inducing activities like watching the news or calling your mother before bed.

## Sip Herbal Tea or Use Other Natural Sleep Remedies

You'd be surprised at how naturally sedating certain types of herbal tea can be. I'm not necessarily talking chamomile, though that works for some! If you really can't sleep, try relaxing or sedating herbs like valerian root or kava kava, or an herbal tea like Celestial Seasonings' Sleepytime Tea. Some of these herbal teas may have side effects, however, like next-day drowsiness. If you experience this or another side effect, drinking herbal tea may not be a good idea.

Another excellent sleep inducer, though not an herb, is the mineral magnesium. Take 400 milligrams prior to bedtime.

However, be aware that if you consistently use these supplements to help you sleep you might have trouble in the long term sleeping without them. Always talk to your physician prior to trying a new supplement.

## Time Your Workouts to Maximize Sleep

Exercise improves your sleep quality—in several ways. First, it increases the overall amount of time you spend asleep at night. Second, it increases the amount of time you spend in slow-wave sleep—the most restorative kind. Third, it boosts the release of growth hormone while you're sleeping. Fourth, it physically tires you out! After you've exercised, your body wants to recover, and sleep is a good way of doing that.

I want to emphasize, too, that exercise also provides significant stress relief and can also dissipate excess cortisol for improved sleep quality.

That said, I caution against exercising at night or close to bed-time. By energizing your body, exercise raises your core body temperature, which is the opposite of what you want to have happen before going to sleep. Your body temperature naturally lowers in the evening, about two hours prior to bedtime, a signal to your brain that it's time to snooze.

So plan your workouts earlier in the day. Studies suggest that working out at 7:00 A.M. or between 1:00 P.M. and 4:00 P.M. could shift the body's clock earlier, helping you fall asleep more easily.

## Practice My Quick Sleep Technique

My technique is a combination of muscle relaxation and deep breathing. It can help you fall asleep in less than five minutes, especially with continued practice. Here's how:

- Lie in bed, on your back (or your most comfortable position for sleep).
- Relax the muscles in your face, including those inside your mouth. You have around forty-three muscles in your face, so they play a huge part in how you destress and prep your body for sleep. Let your whole face—forehead, cheeks, tongue, mouth area, eye area, nose, and jaw—all go slack.
- Drop your shoulders to release tension—picture them falling down to your feet—and let your hands and arms rest at the sides of your body. Let them go slack too.
- Relax your chest muscles as you inhale and exhale.
- Relax the muscles in your thighs and calves—all the muscles in your legs. Let them go limp.
- To clear your mind of worries ("I've got to get the grocery shopping done" or "I must not forget to pay the electric bill"), visualize a scene that is relaxing to you and stay focused on it.

With your muscles and body relaxed, begin to breathe in the following manner:

- Open your lips slightly and exhale through your mouth, making a whooshing sound.
- Close your lips, then slowly inhale through your nose for a count of 4.
- Hold your breath for 7 seconds.
- After, exhale (with a whoosh sound) for 8 seconds.
- Complete this cycle for four full breaths.

Within five minutes, if not sooner, you should be drifting into sleep. A version of this method has been used by the military and was found to help 96 percent of those tested in the U.S. Army to fall asleep within two minutes.

Sleep is king, no one will deny that. It's key to improving just about every aspect of health, including hunger, cravings, even the type of food we choose. When your body gets the right amount of sleep and rest, the decision-making capacity of your brain works at peak performance. You'll stop reaching for chips and cookies (like you do when you're tired) and reach for foods that will truly nourish your mind, body, and spirit.

# 9

## Step 5: Retrain

SHELLY HAD A LOVE-HATE RELATIONSHIP with exercise. Intellectually, she loved the health benefits you can derive from working out. But she hated the idea that exercising might make her hungry—she believed that the more physically active she was, the more her appetite would increase and as a result, she'd eat more and gain weight.

"After all, wouldn't my body want to replace all the calories burned and the nutrients used during a jog or night out dancing?" she asked me.

Because of her conviction, Shelly resisted doing any type of workout that felt hard. She stuck to some moderate walking or some occasional yoga. Because of this, the rush of feel-good chemicals from working out eluded her, and she never really developed an exercise routine she wanted to stick with.

Working with Shelly piqued my interest in whether exercise does make us hungrier and whether it can wreck our weight-loss goals. Because I love to exercise, I wanted to know: Does exercise increase or decrease hunger? What is the real story?

I pored over plenty of studies on this topic, and the answer is: it depends! Studies hint that if you select the right type of exercise—and stick with it—you can actually normalize your hunger levels and your cravings. Which is exactly what I told Shelly—that she had not found the right kind of exercise to control her hunger and cravings.

So the message in this final step is: get moving and you'll stop being so effing hungry! Step 5—Retrain—gives you strategies to make that happen.

## EXERCISE, HUNGER, AND HORMONES

Exercise is much more than a calorie burner; it also influences hormones, neurotransmitters, and other bodily chemicals—and in doing so, it impacts hunger and appetite. Different types of exercise affect our hunger cues differently. I'll explain how this works in this section—take a look!

### Run to Manage Your Hunger Hormones

A study in the *American Journal of Physiology* demonstrated that a sixty-minute run lowered levels of ghrelin (a hormone that stimulates hunger) and raised levels of peptide YY, or PYY (a hormone that suppresses hunger)—both of these signs show that running can tame hunger.

In another study—this one from the University of Wyoming and published in the *Journal of Obesity*—researchers studied a group of women who either ran or walked and, on alternate days, sat quietly for an hour. After the running, walking, or sitting, researchers drew blood samples and analyzed them for levels of certain hormones. They then took the women to a dining room to enjoy a buffet.

From the blood samples, the researchers observed that after the run, the women's ghrelin levels spiked. This should have meant they'd attack the buffet like crazy (as we noted earlier, ghrelin stimulates appetite). But the women did not. In fact, after the run, they ate several hundred fewer calories than they burned off!

Why did this happen? Their restraint, the researchers said, was due to a simultaneous surge in satiety hormones. Those hormones signaled the body that it was adequately fueled, and it was time to stop eating. The escalation of satiety hormones, the authors wrote, muted signals from ghrelin.

Neither sitting nor walking changed the levels of the women's satiety hormones—a situation that triggered them to overeat at the buffet, taking in more calories than they had burned off.

Very interesting, I think! The takeaway is that a good, long run can actually tame your hunger by boosting satiety hormones!

If running sounds like something you'd like to get into, here are a few guidelines on how to start.

Select the right shoes. Running shoes are very specific to the activity—no hiking shoes, cross-trainers, or walking shoes. Running shoes make your runs more enjoyable and help prevent injury.

- Warm up with some light stretching.
- Begin gradually—with up to just 1 minute of running. Alternate with 2 minutes of walking for a total of 20 to 30 minutes. Increase your running time by 30 seconds each week until you reach 10 minutes of running. Increase from there and log your progress.
- Stay hydrated during runs.
- Rest from running on some days during the week so that your body properly recovers.

## Strength Train to Tame Ghrelin

The same study in the *American Journal of Physiology* referenced about running's effect on hormones also revealed that a ninety-minute strength-training workout lowered ghrelin levels, but did not impact PYY. This finding indicates that anaerobic exercise like weight lifting can also suppress appetite but not as much as intense aerobic exercise.

With strength training, exercisers often work out their bodies in "splits," meaning they might train their upper bodies one day, and their lower bodies the next. But according to another study, full-body workouts suppress hunger more than upper/lower splits, even when the training volume is equally intense.

In this study, researchers took twelve recreationally active men with about four years of training experience and put them all through three different workouts, each separated by a washout week.

For the full-body workout, they performed six exercises for three sets each, the last set taken to failure (when your muscles exhaust and you can't lift past a certain poundage).

For the lower-body-only workout, they performed three exercises for six sets each, the last set taken to failure.

For the upper-body-only workout, they again performed three exercises for six sets each, the last set taken to failure.

Using a hunger scale, the researchers measured the men's hunger at multiple points. Ratings were the same after an overnight fast, after breakfast, and before exercising to limit confounding variables. In other words, everyone had the same appetite prior to doing the workouts.

Blood lactate levels, measured in all participants, were strongly correlated with the decreases in hunger. The more lactate that was produced, the less hungry the men were. Lactic acid is a natural chemical produced by muscle tissue and by red blood cells, which transport oxygen from your lungs to other organs of your body. In other studies, it has been found to suppress the secretion of hunger-boosting ghrelin.

All of this makes sense: training more muscle mass creates more lactate, which suppresses appetite. If you want additional appetite-suppressing benefits from strength training, train your full body in one workout.

To start a strength-training program:

- Hire a coach or qualified fitness trainer who can show you the ropes.
- If you like to work out at home, you can find lots of strength-training programs on TV or through streaming services that can guide you through workouts.

- Decide on which exercises to perform to work your entire body in one session.
- Start with poundages you can lift for 15 to 20 reps comfortably for 2 to 3 sets. If the weight feels too light, add 5 to 10 pounds and try again. Once the exercise gets easier, slowly add more weight.
- Work out at least two days a week, for 45 minutes each, on nonconsecutive days to allow your muscles to rest, repair, and develop.
- Stay consistent.

## Do Yoga to Curb Cravings and Choose Healthier Foods

It turns out that a yoga practice is just as good for taming hunger as running and strength training are, but in a couple of different ways. In a study published in 2018 in the *International Journal of Behavioral Nutrition and Physical Activity,* researchers observed that people who do yoga on a regular basis eat less fast food and snacks and eat more fruits and vegetables (which tame hunger and cravings).

Interviews with people in the study revealed that yoga supported nutritious eating because the participants were highly motivated to eat healthy foods, practice greater mindfulness at meals, and manage emotional eating. Plus, they experienced fewer food cravings!

Other research shows that yoga can reduce binge eating by a whopping 51 percent. Experts suggest that yoga works by increasing body awareness (part of the bodyset I talked about on page 69), so you're more sensitive to feeling full and less likely to mindlessly stuff yourself.

Pretty impressive findings, right? Yoga does a lot to help you un-learn unhealthy eating patterns!

To start a yoga practice:

- Choose a type of yoga. There are many different styles of yoga. Hatha is very common and a good choice for beginners. Gyms and fitness centers offer yoga classes, and these are a good starting point. So, of course, are yoga studios.

---

- Watch a few beginner yoga classes online to get a feel for how the movements flow.
- Dress comfortably because yoga involves a lot of stretching.
- Never feel intimidated. Yoga poses can be modified to accommodate beginners.
- Try to practice yoga at least two or three times a week. You'll become more flexible after your very first class. Stay consistent.

## Go Out in Nature to Help with Emotional Overeating

Living in complete harmony with nature, as well as with ourselves, is a large part of Ayurveda. This is why I recommend getting a dose of nature every day—whether it's a quick walk or rolling down the car window on your commute. (Being out in nature resets circadian rhythm too.)

One study I read in *Psychological Science* looked at nature walks versus urban walks and found a significant increase in mood, reduced depression, and higher cognition (brain power) in people who took nature walks versus walking in the city.

Why was one type of walk better than the other?

The researchers concluded that walking in nature calms the brain more effectively, because you don't have to pay as much attention to your surroundings as you would when walking in urban areas.

Let me add here that many people overeat when they're down and depressed. Because exercising in nature lifts moods and eases depressive symptoms, it may help you stop self-medicating with food.

---

### Hunger Hack: Put Some Oomph into Your Workouts

In addition to the type of workout you do, there are other exercise-related issues involved in physical activity and hunger control.

---

## Intensify Your Workouts

A harder workout like an intense spin class tends to dampen appetite, while low- to moderate-intensity exercise like walking can make you feel hungry more quickly. Here's why: During a challenging workout, your body shuttles a lot of blood to the heart, brain, and muscles. Meanwhile, your digestive system gets more or less forgotten. Any food left in there stays for a while and keeps you feeling full. So the more intensely you exercise, the more blood you pull away from the gut and, consequently, the less hungry you'll feel.

## Go Longer

The longer you exercise, the longer it's going to take for your system to return to its resting state and for hunger to kick in. So, after a ninety-minute run, for example, you can jump in the shower, get dressed, and prepare a nice meal before you even feel hungry.

What does all this mean? Although I typically recommend low-intensity workouts for those who are suffering from exhaustion and stress, when you recover, you might want to incrementally increase the intensity and duration of your workouts for better overall craving control. Intense, longer workouts can go a long way toward controlling your appetite, especially when you stay consistent. Strive to work out harder and make it a goal to increase the duration of your exercise sessions.

# HARNESS THE CONNECTION BETWEEN EXERCISE AND NEUROTRANSMITTERS

Exercise and the brain have a tight relationship—so tight, in fact, that exercise dramatically improves mood, mental health, and even hunger and cravings.

What exactly is going on? Simply put, alterations occur in brain biochemistry when you get moving—primarily in the neurotransmitters.

There are three key neurotransmitters involved in hunger, appetite, and exercise: serotonin, dopamine, and GABA. You can use your workouts to activate all three—and normalize hunger and cravings without one lick of willpower.

## Boost Serotonin with Exercise

You've heard of, or experienced, the euphoric feeling some people get when exercising (runner's high, for example). This feeling has been attributed to endorphins, natural feel-good, pain-killing chemicals in the body. There is, however, no strong research to prove endorphins are fully responsible for this feeling. More than likely, serotonin provides that uplifting rush during exercise.

Through lots of research, we know that exercise definitely increases the brain's production of serotonin, which is associated with mood, appetite, and libido. An article published in the *Journal of Psychiatry and Neuroscience* included exercise among the several natural approaches to boosting serotonin levels in the brain. We also know that serotonin is an appetite suppressant, and low levels of this neurotransmitter can trigger cravings for carbs.

Are some forms of exercise better than others for boosting serotonin?

Honestly, almost any exercise or physical activity will do it, but aerobic, cardio-based exercise is particularly beneficial. Although duration is important, as little as fifteen to twenty minutes of movement such as running, jogging, swimming, biking, or working out on a stair-stepper can trigger a serotonin surge and generate a major mood boost.

If you can do your cardio outdoors, all the better. Being outside in the sun stimulates your body's production of serotonin. The sun's ultraviolet rays help your skin absorb vitamin D, which assists the body in manufacturing serotonin. So to get a powerful mood boost, use your outdoor time for working out. Go for a run, jog, hike, or bike ride to churn out more serotonin through both exercise and the absorption of vitamin D.

I also suggest yoga for a serotonin boost. If you're feeling down or anxious, yoga can help by elevating serotonin and reducing stress. In a study published in the *Journal of Alternative and Complementary Medicine*, researchers found that yoga not only increased serotonin, it also reduced excess adrenaline (a stress hormone) and increased levels of antioxidants and immune-boosting chemicals in the body.

## Use Dopamine to Motivate Your Workouts

Hate exercise? Don't blame yourself, blame your brain!

Dopamine drives your motivation to move. So if you can't seem to get off your couch and out the door to the gym, the reason may run deeper than a simple dislike of exercise. A lack of dopamine could be holding you back.

But here's a catch-22: exercise itself boosts the release of dopamine. To capitalize on that fact, put the proverbial cart before the horse and form a workout habit before your motivation kicks in. People who work out habitually know how good they feel post exercise, and one reason is that dopamine is already surging in their brains. To achieve the same, get in a regular workout routine to start enjoying the feel-good effects of dopamine.

However, you don't need to go whole hog on some super-intense workout routines to start feeling more motivated. You can build up with lower-intensity exercise until your workout habit is solidified. Try walking, yoga, or other low-impact exercises to increase dopamine levels. One benefit of sticking with an exercise routine is that it creates daily habits that keep the dopamine pumping and foster a healthy athletic mindset of setting a goal and achieving it.

Let me add, too, that dopamine gets your competitive juices flowing—which provides that competitive thrill. So if you love running in marathons, playing pick-up games of basketball, or participating in any other sports, you've chosen good activities for yourself if they give you that I-did-it lift when you win or accomplish some sort of athletic goal.

If you're not the athletic type, try seeking out workouts you'll look forward to. Maybe it's time to sign up for a dance class, go paddleboarding or kayaking, or hit the hiking trail. If, as a kid, you loved riding your bike, why not invest in a new set of wheels and start cycling? By choosing to engage in fun workouts, you develop habits that ultimately help set dopamine in motion.

Here's something else that's important to know about dopamine and exercise. Remember that dopamine is a reward chemical that stimulates pleasure. If you go to the gym to lift weights or run on the treadmill, because you think you have to, and you grit your teeth, powering through your workout and looking at the clock, you might not be getting much pleasure from the workout. It's work, not enjoyment. Under those conditions, your body won't release that much dopamine. Dopamine release depends on engagement in pleasurable activities.

But if you layer in pleasurable activities to your workout, like listening to music, doing aerobic dance to music, or exercising in nature, these experiences will accentuate the release of dopamine. Never make your workouts feel like torture or drudgery, but instead think of them as a rewarding labor of love. In doing so, you'll tap into the power of dopamine, plus reap all the amazing fitness benefits of regular exercise.

## Boost GABA

I call GABA (gamma-aminobutyric acid) the brakes of the brain. It is a calming neurotransmitter that lowers the activity of cells in the brain and central nervous system. This moves the brain and the body into lower gear, promoting better sleep, less mental and physical stress, and a calm mood. It can also prevent psychological causes of overindulging and overeating since people with GABA deficiency often eat too much and too fast to cope with their anxiety and stress.

If you struggle with cravings or overeating, or feel overwhelmed or stressed out, you can positively influence GABA levels in your system by:

- Destressing with meditation or yoga. Many studies have shown that meditation and meditative movement practices like yoga or tai chi have scientifically confirmed benefits, including increasing GABA.
- Staying active to boost GABA. In addition to its well-known stress-relief benefits, regular exercise helps to increase GABA and its positive action in the brain.

## What Is the Best Workout for You?

When it comes to exercise, some people are dopamine-wired; others need a serotonin or GABA boost. Take this brief quiz to see how you're wired—and what type of exercise might be best fit for your brain and body in order to help you with hunger and cravings. Circle the response that describes you.

1. I'm extremely motivated.

    Yes

    No

2. I need more motivation.

    Yes

    No

3. I enjoy competition with others.

    Yes

    No

4. I need to relax and chill out more.

    Yes

    No

5. I love to set goals and accomplish them.

    Yes

    No

6. I often feel burned out by stress.

    Yes

    No

7. I like to play games and sports.

 Yes

 No

8. My body feels tense a lot of the time.

 Yes

 No

9. I love adventure.

 Yes

 No

10. I prefer mostly solitary activities.

 Yes

 No

*Scoring*

Look over your answers.

If you circled yes for most of the odd-numbered statements, you are dopamine-wired, which means you'll benefit most from challenging activities with clear and measurable outcomes, such as team sports, track events, skiing, and group fitness classes. These activities are best suited to anyone who is generally exteroceptive, or responds well to stimuli from the environment outside the body.

If you answered yes to most of the even-numbered statements, your best choices are serotonin- and GABA-producing exercises, such as yoga, tai chi, and any noncompetitive outdoor activity or other practice in which performance is not evaluated. These are examples of interoceptive activities, in which you tend to sense the internal workings of your body, such as breath regulation, flexibility, digestion, and so forth.

## Hunger Hack: Time Your Meals and Workouts

Here are some research-based tips to help you normalize your appetite with exercise. A review study published in *Physiology and Behavior* looked at studies on exercise timing and appetite control. Their review noted if you exercise:

- Prior to a meal, you promote weight loss, achieve better weight control, reduce fat accumulation around your belly.
- Right before a meal, you'll feel fuller, reduce your hunger, and lower levels of appetite-stimulating ghrelin.
- In the morning, you can reduce your appetite for the rest of the day.

The bottom line? Timing your meals and workouts is a great hunger tamer.

## **Cravings Crusher:** Diversify Your Gut Microbiome with Exercise

Want another reason to exercise? You'll build a better gut! No, I'm not talking about six-pack abs—I'm talking about your microbiome.

Exercise can build the diversity of your microbiome, so that there are more good bacteria in relation to bad bacteria, and we know that this helps curb cravings and hunger. In research from the University of Illinois, and published in *Medicine and Science in Sports and Exercise*, researchers found that exercising for just six weeks can diversify the population of your microbiome—independent of other factors.

In this study, thirty-two sedentary adults were recruited and samples were taken of their gut bacteria. Next, the participants performed a cardio routine for thirty to sixty minutes three times a week for six weeks. At the end of the six weeks, the researchers took gut samples again.

They discovered that the participants' microbiomes had changed. Many of the participants had an increase in certain beneficial gut microbes that help produce short-chain fatty acids. These fatty acids cut the risk of inflammation, as well as type 2 diabetes, obesity, and heart disease. They also stimulate the secretion of hunger-regulating hormones, such as peptide YY (PYY) and glucagon-like-peptide-1 (GLP-1), which both decrease appetite and make you feel full after eating.

After the initial period of six weeks, the participants were then sedentary for another six weeks. The researchers sampled participants' microbiomes at the end of the sedentary period and found that the good gut bugs had fallen to the levels where they were prior to the experimental exercise period. This finding suggests that the impact of exercise on the microbiome for a period of just six weeks may be transient and that exercise needs to be done regularly for ideal gut diversity.

## ADDITIONAL TIPS: HOW TO PLAN HUNGER-CONTROLLING WORKOUTS

There is more research to be done on exercise and appetite, but there's enough information available to help you plan your workouts to curb hunger and cravings. Some general suggestions:

- Include cardio activity in your weekly routine. It reins in hunger hormones and increases serotonin to help you fight cravings. Thirty minutes of cardio two or three times a week is a good start.
- Consider strength training, perhaps twice a week, and work your entire body each time.
- Fit in some yoga at least twice a week, especially if you're prone to stress or emotional eating or you are low in serotonin.

- Take your workouts outdoors when you can. Exercising in nature effectively controls hunger and cravings—plus, it's pleasurable (good for a dopamine boost!).
- Identify physical activities you enjoy or make them as enjoyable as possible—again to enhance the release of dopamine.

No matter what exercise you pick, all I ask is that you don't base your choices solely on how well they control your hunger. We all need to do cardio, strength-training, and flexibility exercises on a regular basis because they have so many different health benefits. Above all, choose activities that you enjoy so you're more likely to stick with them over the long term.

# Part III

~~~~~~~~~~~~~~~~

# Effing Hungry No More!

# 10

# Incredibly Filling Meals: Reset Your Hunger and Cravings in Two Weeks

**R**EADY TO START TAMING YOUR hunger and crushing your cravings—naturally and automatically? Over the next two weeks, you'll do exactly that, and you'll experience what it feels like to not be so effing hungry!

Each day of meals features foods known to build health plus effortlessly help you feel full and satisfied. Feel free to follow this plan exactly as written or switch around some of the breakfasts, lunches, and dinners. I've also provided examples of when you can use leftovers to avoid wasting food.

Shopping lists follow the meal plan, and the recipes are found in Chapter 11. Here are some additional guidelines to help you.

1. You do not need to follow the meal plan exactly. For example, if your favorite breakfast is one of my smoothies, feel free to enjoy them several days in a row for breakfast. Use the recipes you like best when planning your meals.

2. Each recipe contains hunger tamers and cravings crushers, so try to include as many recipes as possible in your meal planning each day.

3. Eat until you are satisfied, not stuffed.
4. If you choose to do circadian fasting, use your bedtime as a rough marker for timing your meals. You might have your first meal (breakfast) at 10 A.M., for example, and finish your dinner by 8 P.M. You can also shorten your feeding window and lengthen your fasting window by finishing your dinner by 5 P.M. Whatever times you set for your meals, be sure to stop eating two to three hours prior to bedtime.
5. Eat your meals at regular times to control hunger and cravings. It's also a good idea to supplement your meals with raw vegetables or mixed greens, spices, teas, and berries. There is no limit to eating these foods; enjoy them whenever you like.
6. Try to eat a probiotics like yogurt, kefir, or kombucha daily.
7. Stay hydrated. Drink 80 to 100 ounces of water daily.
8. Practice my 3-2-1 technique three times a week.
9. Supplement your day with the three S's—sunlight (at least twenty minutes daily), sleep, and stress relief.

# WEEK 1

## Day 1

Breakfast: High-Fiber Vegan Banana Pancakes with Blueberry Sauce (see page 172)
Lunch: Black Bean and Sweet Potato Hash (see page 182)
Snack: Yogurt Ranch Veggie Dip with raw veggies (see page 193)
Dinner: Date-Olive Chicken/Tofu with Sautéed Kale (see page 179)

## Day 2

Breakfast: Spicy Indian Eggs (see page 173)
Lunch: Leftover Date-Olive Chicken with Sautéed Kale (see page 179)

Snack: Leftover Yogurt Ranch Veggie Dip with raw veggies
(see page 193)

Dinner: Leftover Black Bean and Sweet Potato Hash
(see page 182)

## Day 3

Breakfast: Sweet Cherry–Almond Butter Smoothie
(see page 198)

Lunch: Kimchi (see page 192) with Leek, Cabbage, and Sweet
Potato Soup (see page 194)

Snack: Coconut Kefir with a handful of walnuts (see page 196)

Dinner: Stir-Fry with Tofu, Broccoli, Snow Peas, and Bean
Sprouts (see page 183)

## Day 4

Breakfast: Chai Latte Oatmeal Bowl (see page 175)

Lunch: Leftover Stir-Fry with Tofu, Broccoli, Snow Peas, and
Bean Sprouts (see page 183)

Snack: Cup of leftover Leek, Cabbage, and Sweet Potato Soup
(see page 194)

Dinner: Spiced Moroccan Lentils (see page 189)

## Day 5

Breakfast: Chickpea Omelet with Spinach and Goat Cheese
(see page 176)

Lunch: Crispy Air-Fried Tofu Lettuce Wraps (see page 184)

Snack: Coconut Kefir with a handful of walnuts (see page 196)

Dinner: Leftover Spiced Moroccan Lentils (see page 189)

## Day 6

Breakfast: Turmeric Egg White Scramble with Kale, Chickpeas,
Sweet Potatoes, and Yogurt (see page 177)

Lunch: Creamy Broccoli-Cheese Soup (see page 195)
Snack: Iced Oat Milk Chai (see page 197)
Dinner: Roasted Tempeh and Broccoli with Peanut Sauce
(see page 188)

## Day 7

Breakfast: Mixed Berry Compote with Yogurt (see page 178)
Lunch: Leftover Creamy Broccoli-Cheese Soup
(see page 195)
Snack: Peppermint-Mocha Sipper with a handful of walnuts
(see page 198)
Dinner: Crispy Berbere-Roasted Tofu and Vegetables
(see page 185)

# WEEK 2

## Day 1

Breakfast: Healthiest Yogurt Parfait (see page 178)
Lunch: Leftover Crispy Berbere-Roasted Tofu and Vegetables
(see page 185)
Snack: Dark Chocolate–Dipped Fruit (see page 200)
Dinner: Pan-Seared Salmon with Lemon-Garlic Butter
(see page 191) (this will include the Brussels sprouts
side dish)

## Day 2

Breakfast: Vanilla Chai Protein Shake (see page 197)
Lunch: Lebanese Chopped Kale Salad with Air-Fried Falafel
(see page 181)
Snack: Yogurt Ranch Veggie Dip (see page 193)
Dinner: Garlicky Baby Bok Choy and Shiitake Mushroom
Stir-Fry with Shrimp (see page 191)

# Day 3

Breakfast: High-Protein Oat Pudding with Cardamom and Plums (see page 174)

Lunch: Black Bean and Sweet Potato Hash (see page 182)

Snack: Kombucha (see page 199) with Dark Chocolate–Peppermint Coins with Cacao Nibs (see page 201)

Dinner: Leek, Cabbage, and Sweet Potato Soup with Beef (see page 196)

# Day 4

Breakfast: Spicy Indian Eggs (see page 173)

Lunch: Leftover Leek, Cabbage, and Sweet Potato Soup with Beef (see page 196)

Snack: Sweet Cherry–Almond Butter Smoothie (see page 198)

Dinner: Pan-Seared Salmon with Lemon-Garlic Butter (see page 191) with Kimchi (see page 192)

# Day 5

Breakfast: High-Fiber Vegan Banana Pancakes with Blueberry Sauce (see page 172)

Lunch: Crispy Air-Fried Tofu Lettuce Wraps (see page 184)

Snack: Dark Chocolate–Peppermint Coins with Cacao Nibs (see page 201) with Kombucha (see page 199)

Dinner: Date-Olive Chicken with Sautéed Kale (see page 179)

# Day 6

Breakfast: Pumpkin Spice Chia Seed Pudding (see page 203)

Lunch: Crispy Berbere-Roasted Tofu and Vegetables (see page 185)

Snack: Fudgy Black Bean Brownies (see page 202)

Dinner: Curried Tofu Scramble with Spinach and Tomatoes (see page 186)

## Day 7

Breakfast: Green Tea Yogurt Bowl with Berries and Chocolate
(see page 203)
Lunch: Leftover Curried Tofu Scramble with Spinach and
Tomatoes (see page 186)
Snack: Leftover Fudgy Black Bean Brownies (see page 202)
Dinner: Spiced Moroccan Lentils (see page 189)

After reading over the meal plans and the corresponding recipes,
check the contents of your kitchen and pantry to see what ingredients you already have and which you'll need to shop for. Purchasing
groceries ahead of time will let you prep and cook in advance for
additional convenience.

The shopping lists that follow include all of the ingredients found
in the recipes in Chapter 11. Where quantities are specified, they
are only general guidelines. You may require more or less of certain
foods, depending on how many people you're cooking for and which
recipes you'll be using.

## STAPLES TO HAVE ON HAND

### BAKING NEEDS
Baking powder
Chickpea flour
Cornstarch or arrowroot powder
Nutritional yeast
Unsweetened cocoa powder
White whole wheat flour or gluten-free all-purpose flour

### SPICES AND FLAVORINGS
Aleppo pepper (optional)
Allspice, ground
Berbere seasoning (Ethiopian spice blend)

Black pepper, freshly ground
Cardamom, ground
Cayenne
Chili powder
Cinnamon
Cloves, ground
Coriander, ground
Cumin, ground
Curry powder
Dill, dried
Garam masala
Garlic powder
Ginger, ground
Gochugaru (Korean red chili powder)
Hibiscus petals, dried
Lavender flowers, dried
Onion flakes, dried
Onion powder
Parsley flakes, dried
Peppermint oil
Pumpkin pie spice
Pure vanilla extract
Red pepper flakes
Sea salt
Sea salt, flaked variety
Smoked paprika
Thyme, dried
Turmeric, ground

## CONDIMENTS
Apple cider vinegar
Fish sauce or vegan fish sauce
Red wine vinegar
Low-sodium soy sauce or tamari
Sriracha

## FATS AND OILS
    Almond butter
    Butter
    Coconut oil
    Extra-virgin olive oil
    Ghee
    Mayonnaise
    Peanut butter, natural, creamy
    Sesame oil
    Vegan butter
    Walnut oil

## SWEETENERS
    Agave syrup
    Brown sugar, small amount
    Granulated sugar
    Liquid stevia
    Maple syrup

# WEEK 1 SHOPPING LIST

## FRUIT
    Avocado, 1
    Banana, 1
    Blueberries, fresh or frozen
    Dark sweet cherries, frozen
    Lemons, 2
    Limes, 3
    Orange juice, 3 tablespoons
    Strawberries, frozen
    Raspberries, frozen

## VEGETABLES AND FRESH HERBS
    Baby spinach, 5 ounces
    Bean sprouts, 1 cup

Bibb lettuce leaves, 16 leaves from 1 head
Broccoli, 3 small heads plus broccoli florets, enough for 1½ cups
Cabbage, 10½ cups shredded or pre-shredded cabbage, 14- to
    16-ounce bag
Carrots, 4
Cauliflower florets, 2 cups
Chives, small package
Cilantro, 1 small bunch
Crushed tomatoes, 15-ounce can
Daikon radish, 1
Garlic cloves, 8
Ginger root, 1
Jalapeño pepper, 1
Kale, curly leaf, ½ bunch
Kale, 1 bunch
Leeks, 3 medium
Napa cabbage, 1 medium head
Parsley, 1 bunch
Plum tomato, 1
Red bell pepper, 1
Red onions, 3 small
Rosemary, several sprigs
Russet potato, 1
Scallions, 5
Serrano chili pepper, 2
Shallot, 1
Snow peas, 1 cup
Sweet potatoes, 3 medium, 1 small
Yellow onions, 1 medium, 1 small

PROTEINS

Black beans, 1 15-ounce can
Boneless, skinless chicken breasts, 2
Chickpeas, 1 15-ounce can

Eggs, 4

Liquid egg whites, ½ cup, or whites from 4 eggs, or vegan eggs

Salmon, 4 fillets

Tempeh, 8 ounces

Tofu, 3 14-ounce blocks, extra-firm

Unsweetened plant-based vanilla protein powder, 1 32-ounce canister, such as Orgain Organic Plant-Based Protein Powder

Whole brown or green lentils, 1 cup

BREAD AND GRAINS

Old-fashioned rolled oats

Whole-grain naan

NUTS AND SEEDS

Chia seeds

Flaxseeds, ground

Sesame seeds

Walnuts

DAIRY AND NON-DAIRY FOODS

Buttermilk powder

Coconut, full fat, 2 13.5-ounce cans

Greek yogurt or plant-based yogurt, 2 cups

Oat milk, 1¾ cups

Plant-based milk, any type, unsweetened, 1¼ cups

Sharp cheddar cheese, 4 ounces, grated

Soft goat cheese, 4 ounces; feta cheese crumbles, 4 ounces; or vegan cheese of choice, 4 ounces

MISCELLANEOUS

AmyMD Chai Latte Powder or any chai spice blend (see the recipe on page 175)

Capers

Chicken broth, 4 cups

Dates, pitted

Espresso or strong-brewed coffee

Kalamata olives, pitted, ¼ cup
Kefir starter

# WEEK 2 SHOPPING LIST

FRUIT

Apple, dried, 8 pieces
Apricots, dried, 8
Avocado, 1
Banana, 2
Blackberries, fresh
Blueberries, fresh
Blueberries, 1 cup frozen
Dark sweet cherries, frozen
Lemons, 3
Lime, 1
Orange, 1
Plum, 1 small
Prunes, 8
Raspberries, ½ cup fresh
Strawberries, fresh

VEGETABLES

Baby bok choy, 1 pound
Baby spinach, 1 5-ounce package
Bibb lettuce leaves, 16, from 1 head
Brussels sprouts, 2 pounds
Cabbage, 10½ cups shredded or pre-shredded cabbage, 14- to
    16- ounce bag
Carrots, 6
Cauliflower florets, 4 cups
Cherry or grape tomatoes, ½ cup
Chives
Cilantro, 1 bunch
Crushed tomatoes, 1 15-ounce can

Garlic cloves, 14
Jalapeño pepper, 1
Kale, 1 bunch stems
Leeks, 3 medium
Parsley, 1 bunch
Plum tomato, 1 large
Pumpkin puree, 1 cup
Red bell pepper, 1
Red onions, 6
Rosemary, a few springs
Scallions, 3
Serrano chili pepper, 1
Shallot, 1
Shiitake mushrooms, 4 ounces
Sweet potatoes, 3 medium
Yellow onion, 1 small

PROTEINS
Black beans, 2 15-ounce cans
Boneless, skinless chicken breasts, 2
Eggs, 4
Vegan eggs
Salmon, 8 5- to 6-ounce fillets
Shrimp, medium, 1 pound shelled and deveined
Sirloin, 8 ounces
Tofu, 3 14-ounce blocks, extra firm, plus 1 8-ounce block, extra firm
Unsweetened plant-based vanilla protein powder, 1 32-ounce canister, such as Orgain Organic Plant-Based Protein Powder
Whole brown or green lentils, 1 cup

BREAD AND GRAINS
No-sugar-added granola, ½ cup
Old-fashioned rolled oats, 1 cup
Quick oats, ½ cup
Whole-grain naan

## NUTS AND SEEDS

Almonds
Chia seeds
Flaxseeds, ground
Pecans
Pepitas (pumpkin seeds)
Pistachios
Sesame seeds
Walnuts

## DAIRY AND NON-DAIRY FOODS

Buttermilk powder
Feta cheese crumbles, ¼ cup
Greek yogurt or plant-based yogurt, 4 cups
Oat milk, 1 cup
Plant-based milk, any type, unsweetened, 5 cups

## MISCELLANEOUS

AmyMD Chai Latte Powder or any chai spice blend (see the
  recipe on page 175)
Cacao nibs
Capers
Chicken or vegetable broth, 2½ cups
Dates, pitted
High-quality matcha powder
Kalamata olives, pitted, ¼ cup
SCOBY (symbiotic culture of bacteria and yeast), 1 (see the
  sourcing note on page 200)
Starter liquid, 1 to 2 cups
Sugar-free dark chocolate chips, 24 ounces, plus ½ cup
Tea bags (green, black, white, or a combination), 6

# 11

# Delicious Recipes That Keep You Full

Now it's time to get cooking! The following recipes are a compilation of the most hunger-taming—plus super-delicious—dishes you can find and many are inspired by my cultural heritage. Most are vegan or vegetarian, but feel free to sub in organically raised fish, chicken, or beef where desired.

All the recipes follow my guidelines for taming hunger and crushing cravings, and feature the foods I've highlighted in this book. I've labeled the recipes that are cravings crushers (CC) and hunger tamers (HT) as well as those that are vegan (V) and gluten-free (GF). Each recipe has been designed to work hand in hand with my meal plan.

Enjoy!

# BREAKFAST/BRUNCH DISHES

## High-Fiber Vegan Banana Pancakes with Blueberry Sauce

*V, GF, CC*

*Makes 2 to 4 servings*

FOR THE PANCAKES

    1 cup white whole wheat flour or gluten-free all-purpose flour
    2 tablespoons ground flaxseed
    2 teaspoons baking powder
    ¼ teaspoon sea salt
    ½ teaspoon cinnamon
    1 large ripe banana, mashed until almost liquefied
    1 cup oat milk
    ½ teaspoon pure vanilla extract
    1 tablespoon maple syrup or 6 to 9 drops liquid stevia (optional)
    Vegan butter, for frying

FOR THE BLUEBERRY SAUCE

    1 cup fresh or frozen blueberries
    ¼ cup plus 1 tablespoon water
    ¼ cup pure maple syrup or ½ teaspoon liquid stevia
    1 tablespoon fresh lemon juice
    1 tablespoon cornstarch or arrowroot powder
    ¼ teaspoon pure vanilla extract
    1½ teaspoons lemon zest

1. For the pancakes: In a medium bowl, whisk together the flour, flaxseed, baking powder, salt, and cinnamon. Make a well in the center.
2. In a small bowl, whisk together the banana, oat milk, vanilla, and maple syrup (if using). Pour the liquid ingredients into the dry ingredients all at once. Gently stir just until blended. The batter will be a little lumpy—that's okay. Let stand for 10 minutes.
3. Meanwhile, make the blueberry sauce: In a small saucepan, combine the blueberries, ¼ cup water, maple syrup, and lemon juice. Bring to a low boil, stirring frequently. In a small bowl,

whisk together the cornstarch and 1 tablespoon cold or room temperature water. Slowly add to the blueberries, stirring constantly. Simmer until the sauce coats the back of a spoon, about 5 minutes. Remove from the heat and stir in vanilla and lemon zest. Set aside.

4. To cook the pancakes, melt some butter in a large nonstick skillet over medium heat. When the butter bubbles, scoop ¼-cup spoonfuls of batter into the pan. Cook the pancakes until bubbles appear on the surface and the underside is golden brown. Flip and cook until golden brown on the other side. Repeat with the remaining batter, adding more butter as needed.

5. Serve immediately, topped with warm blueberry sauce.

## Spicy Indian Eggs

*GF (if naan is not eaten), V (if vegan eggs are used), HT*
*Makes 2 servings*

1 tablespoon ghee, butter, or vegan butter
½ small red onion, finely chopped
1 serrano chili pepper, seeded and finely chopped
1 clove garlic, minced
¼ teaspoon ground cumin
¼ teaspoon garam masala
¼ teaspoon ground turmeric
Sea salt
1 large plum tomato, seeded and finely chopped
4 eggs, beaten, or 4 vegan eggs
¼ cup chopped fresh cilantro, divided
Whole-grain naan, toasted, for serving (optional)

1. Melt the ghee in a medium nonstick skillet over medium-low heat. Add the onion, chili pepper, and garlic. Cook, stirring frequently, until onion is softened, about 5 minutes. Add the cumin, garam masala, turmeric, and salt to taste. Cook, stirring frequently, until the spices are aromatic.

2. Add the tomato and cook, stirring gently, for 1 minute. Add the eggs and reduce heat to low. Cook, stirring occasionally,

until the eggs are cooked through but still glossy, about 5 minutes. Stir in half of the cilantro and remove the skillet from the heat. Allow to stand for 1 minute, stirring once, until the eggs are set.

3. Divide between two plates and sprinkle with the remaining cilantro. Serve with toasted naan, if desired.

## High-Protein Oat Pudding with Cardamom and Plums

*V, GF, HT*

*Makes 1 serving*

½ cup old-fashioned rolled oats
1 cup unsweetened plant-based milk, divided
¾ cup water
¼ teaspoon ground cardamom, divided
Pinch sea salt
1 scoop unsweetened plant-based vanilla protein powder
1 tablespoon almond butter
2 tablespoons Greek yogurt or plant-based yogurt
2 teaspoons pure maple syrup or 6 drops liquid stevia, divided
1 small ripe plum, pitted and chopped, or ½ cup sliced fresh strawberries

1. In a small saucepan, combine the oats, ¾ cup of the milk, the water, ⅛ teaspoon of the cardamom, and salt. Bring to a boil then reduce the heat. Simmer until the oats are tender, about 4 minutes. Transfer the oats to a bowl; allow to cool slightly. Stir in the protein powder, remaining ¼ cup milk, almond butter, yogurt, and 1 teaspoon of the maple syrup (or 3 drops of the stevia). Let cool completely, then cover and chill overnight.

2. To serve, toss the plum, remaining ⅛ teaspoon cardamom, and remaining 1 teaspoon maple syrup (or 3 drops stevia) in a small bowl. Let stand 5 minutes.

3. Top the pudding with the fruit and accumulated juices and serve.

# Chai Latte Oatmeal Bowl

*V, GF, HT*

*Makes 2 servings*

FOR THE OATMEAL

2 cups water

¼ teaspoon sea salt

1 cup old-fashioned rolled oats

2 scoops AmyMD Chai Latte Powder (see Note) or chai spice blend (recipe follows)

1 teaspoon pure vanilla extract

½ cup unsweetened plant-based milk (plain or vanilla)

FOR THE TOPPINGS

Unsweetened coconut chips, lightly toasted

Flaxseeds

Fresh berries, such as strawberries, raspberries, blueberries, and/or blackberries

1. In a small saucepan, bring the water and salt to a boil over medium-high heat. Reduce the heat to a simmer and stir in the oats and Chai Latte Powder. Cook, stirring frequently, until the oats are thick and creamy, about 10 minutes.
2. Remove the saucepan from the heat and stir in the vanilla extract and plant-based milk.
3. Divide the oatmeal between two bowls and top with coconut chips, flaxseeds, and fresh berries.

Note: If you don't have AmyMD Chai Latte Powder on hand, stir in ½ teaspoon of a store-bought chai spice blend and 8 drops liquid stevia with the vanilla extract and plant-based milk. Alternatively, you can make your own chai spice blend by combining:

¼ to ½ cup instant tea powder

1 teaspoon ground ginger

1 teaspoon ground cinnamon

½ teaspoon ground cardamom

½ teaspoon ground cloves

# Chickpea Omelet with Spinach and Goat Cheese

*V, GF, HT*

*Makes 2 servings*

 1 cup chickpea flour
 2 tablespoons nutritional yeast
 ½ teaspoon baking powder
 ½ teaspoon smoked paprika
 ¼ teaspoon garlic powder
 ¼ teaspoon onion powder
 Sea salt
 3 tablespoons extra-virgin olive oil
 5 ounces baby spinach
 Freshly ground black pepper
 4 ounces soft goat cheese, crumbled feta, or vegan
   cheese of choice

1. In a medium bowl, whisk together the chickpea flour, nutritional yeast, baking powder, smoked paprika, garlic powder, onion powder, and ½ teaspoon salt. Slowly whisk in a scant 1 cup water. Set aside for 10 minutes or up to 1 hour to thicken.
2. While the batter is resting, heat 1 tablespoon of the extra-virgin olive oil in a large nonstick skillet over medium-high heat. Add the spinach and cook, tossing frequently, just until wilted, about 2 minutes. (The spinach should still be bright green.) Carefully drain off the excess liquid. Season to taste with salt and pepper. Set aside.
3. To cook the omelets, heat 1 tablespoon of the olive oil in a medium nonstick skillet over medium-high heat. When the oil is shimmering and almost smoking, swirl the oil around the pan and immediately pour ¾ cup of the chickpea batter into the pan, swirling to coat. Cook undisturbed for 1 minute, until the surface of the omelet looks dry and slides around the pan easily. Cover the surface with half of the spinach and half of the cheese. Cook for 30 seconds, then use a thin spatula to fold the omelet in half. Cook 1 minute more, flipping halfway through,

until the cheese is melted and omelet is golden. Repeat with the remaining 1 tablespoon of oil, batter, spinach, and cheese.

4. Serve immediately.

## Turmeric Egg White Scramble with Kale, Chickpeas, Sweet Potatoes, and Yogurt

*V, GF, HT*

*Makes 2 servings*

1 small sweet potato, peeled and cut into small cubes
2 tablespoons extra-virgin olive oil, divided
Sea salt and freshly ground black pepper
½ bunch curly-leaf kale, stemmed and torn into large pieces
⅔ cup canned chickpeas, drained and rinsed
½ cup liquid egg whites or vegan eggs
¼ teaspoon ground turmeric
½ cup plain Greek yogurt or plant-based yogurt
Aleppo pepper (optional)
Lime wedges, for serving

1. Preheat the oven to 425°F. In a medium bowl, toss the sweet potato with 2 teaspoons of the olive oil and season to taste with salt and pepper. Spread out on half of a large, rimmed baking pan and roast for 20 minutes.

2. After the sweet potatoes have been roasting for 20 minutes, place the kale in a medium bowl and drizzle with 2 teaspoons of the olive oil. Massage gently for 30 seconds to tenderize. Add the chickpeas to the bowl, season to taste with salt and pepper, and toss to combine. Spread the kale and chickpeas on the other half of the baking pan and roast until the kale is lightly browned around the edges and crisp tender, about 5 minutes, and the sweet potatoes are tender and starting to brown and caramelize.

3. Meanwhile, in a medium bowl, whisk the egg whites with the turmeric and add salt and pepper to taste. Lightly season the yogurt with salt. Heat the remaining 2 teaspoons of olive oil in a medium nonstick skillet over medium heat. Add the egg whites

and cook until desired consistency. Add the kale, chickpeas, and sweet potatoes to the skillet and toss to combine.

4. To serve, divide the yogurt between two plates. Top with the egg mixture. Sprinkle with Aleppo pepper, if using, and serve with lime wedges.

## Mixed Berry Compote with Yogurt

*V (if plant-based yogurt is used), GF, HT*
*Makes about 2½ cups of compote*

> 3 cups frozen fruit (strawberries, raspberries, dark sweet cherries, or a combination)
> 3 tablespoons orange juice
> ½ teaspoon grated fresh ginger (or ¼ teaspoon ground)
> 1 teaspoon chia seeds
> ¾ cup plain Greek yogurt or plant-based yogurt, to serve

1. In a small saucepan, bring the fruit, orange juice, and ginger to a boil over medium heat. Reduce the heat and use a wooden spoon to gently mash the fruit.
2. Cook over medium-low for 8 to 10 minutes, stirring occasionally, until the fruit has slightly thickened. Remove from the heat and stir in the chia seeds.
3. Transfer the fruit to a clean jar or container and allow to cool completely. Store in the refrigerator for up to 1 week or freeze in ice cube molds and store frozen for up to 1 month.
4. To serve, spoon the Greek yogurt into a bowl. Swirl in ½ cup of the compote.

## Healthiest Yogurt Parfait

*V (if plant-based yogurt is used), GF, HT*
*Makes 2 servings*

> ½ cup no-sugar-added granola
> ¼ cup sliced almonds, toasted
> 1½ cups plain Greek yogurt or plant-based yogurt

2 tablespoons pure maple syrup or ¼ teaspoon liquid
　　stevia, divided
½ teaspoon pure vanilla extract
2 tablespoons ground flaxseed
½ cup sliced strawberries
½ cup blueberries
½ cup raspberries
1 teaspoon orange zest

1. In a small bowl, stir together the granola and almonds.
2. In another small bowl, stir together the yogurt, 1 tablespoon of
   the maple syrup (or ⅛ teaspoon liquid stevia), vanilla extract,
   and flaxseed.
3. In a third small bowl, stir together the strawberries, blueberries,
   and raspberries. Drizzle with the remaining 1 tablespoon
   of maple syrup (or ⅛ teaspoon liquid stevia), and sprinkle
   with the orange zest. Toss to combine and let stand for 5 to
   10 minutes.
4. Into each of two glasses, scoop ⅓ cup of the yogurt. Top the
   yogurt with some of the fruit, then some granola-nut mixture
   followed by more yogurt, layering until the glasses are almost
   full and ending with fruit and granola. Serve immediately.

# ENTREES

## Date-Olive Chicken/Tofu with Sautéed Kale

*GF, HT*

*Makes 2 servings*

### FOR THE CHICKEN/TOFU
2 boneless, skinless chicken breasts or 1 8-ounce package
　　tempeh, cut in 2 pieces
Sea salt and freshly ground black pepper
1 tablespoon extra-virgin olive oil
½ cup pitted dates, halved
¼ cup pitted Kalamata olives, drained

1 shallot, thinly sliced
¼ cup chicken broth
1 tablespoon red wine vinegar
1 tablespoon capers, drained
1 sprig fresh rosemary

FOR THE KALE
1 tablespoon extra-virgin olive oil
1 clove garlic, thinly sliced
1 bunch kale, stems removed and leaves chopped
¼ cup chicken broth
Sea salt and freshly ground black pepper
Chopped fresh parsley (optional)

1. For the chicken: Preheat the oven to 375°F. Season the chicken to taste with salt and pepper. In a medium oven-proof skillet, heat the olive oil over medium-high heat. Add the chicken and cook until browned, turning once, about 5 minutes.
2. Remove the skillet from the heat. Add the dates, olives, shallots, broth, vinegar, capers, and rosemary to the skillet with the chicken, stirring around the chicken to combine.
3. Transfer the skillet to the oven and roast, uncovered, until the internal temperature of the chicken is 165°F and the chicken is no longer pink, 15 to 18 minutes.
4. Meanwhile, for the kale: In a large skillet, heat the olive oil over medium heat. Add the garlic and cook, stirring, until fragrant, about 30 seconds. Add the kale and broth and stir to combine. Cover and cook until the kale is wilted, about 5 minutes. Uncover and cook, stirring frequently, until all the liquid has evaporated, 2 to 3 minutes. Season to taste with salt and pepper.
5. Divide the kale between two places. Arrange the chicken, dates, and olives on top of the kale. Drizzle all with the pan juices. Sprinkle with parsley, if using.

# Lebanese Chopped Kale Salad with Air-Fried Falafel

*V, GF, HT*

*Makes 4 servings*

### FOR THE TAHINI DRESSING
½ cup tahini
⅔ to ¾ cup water
3 tablespoons fresh lemon juice
1 clove garlic, minced
1 tablespoon extra-virgin olive oil
Sea salt and freshly ground black pepper

### FOR THE SALAD
12 pieces frozen gluten-free falafel
1 small bunch curly-leaf kale, stems removed, chopped
Extra-virgin olive oil
1 large ripe tomato, diced
2 Persian cucumbers (also called mini cucumbers), diced
½ large green pepper, chopped
5 radishes, trimmed and diced
2 scallions, chopped
¼ cup chopped fresh parsley
½ cup Kalamata olives
¼ cup crumbled feta cheese or vegan feta cheese (optional)

1. For the dressing: In a small jar with a lid, combine the tahini, ⅔ cup of the water, lemon juice, garlic, olive oil, and salt and pepper to taste. Shake until well blended, adding more water to achieve desired consistency. Set aside.
2. For the salad: Preheat the air fryer to 375°F for 5 minutes. Layer the falafel in the air fryer basket and cook until crisp and golden brown, about 8 minutes, turning once. (Oven method: Bake at 400°F for 8 to 9 minutes, turning once.)
3. While the falafel is cooking, place the kale in a large bowl. Drizzle with a little olive oil. Massage for 2 to 3 minutes or until tender. Add the tomato, cucumbers, green pepper, radishes, scallions, and parsley. Toss to combine. Drizzle with the desired amount of dressing and toss again.

4. To serve, divide the salad among 4 plates. Sprinkle with olives and feta cheese, if using. Top each salad with 3 pieces of falafel. Drizzle with additional dressing. Serve immediately.

## Black Bean and Sweet Potato Hash

*V, GF, CC*

*Makes 4 servings*

1 tablespoon extra-virgin olive oil
1 small red onion, chopped
1 medium sweet potato, peeled and cut into ½-inch dice
2 cloves garlic, minced
1 jalapeño chili pepper, seeded and minced
2 teaspoons ground cumin
2 teaspoons chili powder
¾ cup chicken broth or water
1 15-ounce can black beans, rinsed and drained
2 tablespoons chopped fresh cilantro
Sea salt and freshly ground black pepper
1 avocado, peeled, pitted, and diced
Lime wedges

1. In a large skillet, heat the olive oil over medium-high heat. Add the onion and cook, stirring frequently, until lightly browned in spots, about 3 to 4 minutes. Add the sweet potato and cook, stirring frequently, until it starts to brown in spots, about 5 to 7 minutes.
2. Stir in the garlic, jalapeño, cumin, and chili powder. Cook, stirring frequently, until fragrant, about 30 seconds. Add the chicken broth and cook, scraping up any browned bits, until the liquid is evaporated, 3 to 5 minutes.
3. Stir in the black beans and cook until heated through. Stir in the cilantro and season to taste with salt and pepper. Top with the diced avocado and serve with lime wedges.

# Stir-Fry with Tofu, Broccoli, Snow Peas, and Bean Sprouts

*V, GF, HT, CC*

*Makes 4 servings*

> 1 14-ounce block extra-firm tofu
> ¼ cup low-sodium soy sauce or tamari
> 3 tablespoons rice wine vinegar
> 3 tablespoons sesame oil, divided, plus more if needed
> 2 cloves garlic, minced
> 2 teaspoons grated fresh ginger
> 1 teaspoon maple syrup or 2 drops liquid stevia
> Pinch of red pepper flakes (optional)
> 1 tablespoon cornstarch or arrowroot powder
> 1½ cups broccoli florets
> 1 cup snow peas, trimmed and strings removed
> 1 cup fresh bean sprouts
> 2 scallions, trimmed and sliced

1. Line a plate with two layers of paper towels. Place the tofu on the paper towels. Top with two additional layers of paper towels. Set a heavy skillet on top of the tofu and let stand for 15 minutes to press and drain off excess liquid. Cut the tofu into ½-inch cubes. Set aside.

2. In a small bowl, whisk together the soy sauce, rice wine vinegar, 1 tablespoon of the sesame oil, garlic, ginger, maple syrup, and red pepper flakes, if using. Remove half of the sauce (about ¼ cup) and drizzle it over the tofu, tossing to coat. Let stand 15 minutes. Whisk the cornstarch into the remaining sauce and set aside.

3. In a nonstick wok or large skillet, heat the remaining 2 tablespoons sesame oil over medium-high heat. Add the marinated tofu and cook, stirring occasionally, until golden brown. Remove from the pan.

4. Add more oil to the pan, if necessary. Add the broccoli and cook, stirring frequently, for 2 to 3 minutes. Add the snow peas and cook, stirring frequently, for 1 to 2 minutes. Add the bean sprouts and cook, stirring frequently, for 1 to 2 minutes. Return

the tofu to the pan along with the reserved sauce. Cook and stir until bubbling and slightly thickened, 1 to 2 minutes.

5. Divide the stir-fry among 4 plates. Sprinkle with the scallions and serve.

## Crispy Air-Fried Tofu Lettuce Wraps

V, GF, CC
*Makes 4 servings (2 wraps each)*

**FOR THE TOFU**
- 1 14-ounce block extra-firm tofu
- 2 tablespoons low-sodium soy sauce
- 2 tablespoons sesame oil
- 1 clove garlic, minced

**FOR THE SLAW**
- 1 tablespoon rice vinegar
- 2 teaspoons low-sodium soy sauce
- 1 teaspoon pure maple syrup or 3 to 4 drops liquid stevia
- 1 teaspoon sesame oil
- 2 teaspoons grated fresh ginger
- 2½ cups shredded cabbage (red, green, or a mix)
- ½ cup shredded carrot
- ½ red bell pepper, very thinly sliced
- 1 scallion, thinly sliced
- 2 tablespoons chopped fresh cilantro

**FOR SERVING**
- ½ cup good-quality mayonnaise
- ½ to 1 teaspoon sriracha
- 16 Bibb lettuce leaves
- 1 teaspoon sesame seeds, toasted

1. For the tofu: Line a plate with two layers of paper towels. Place the tofu on the paper towels. Top with two additional layers of paper towels. Set a heavy skillet on top of the tofu and let stand for 15 minutes to press and drain off excess liquid. Cut the tofu into 16 rectangular blocks.

2. Place the tofu in a large bowl. In a small bowl, whisk together the soy sauce, sesame oil, and garlic. Drizzle the marinade over the tofu and toss gently to coat. Let marinate for 15 minutes.

3. Preheat the air fryer to 375°F for 5 minutes. Arrange the tofu in the air fryer basket in a single layer. Cook for 10 to 15 minutes, turning halfway through the cooking time, until the tofu is browned and crispy. (Oven method: Bake at 400°F for 12 to 15 minutes, turning once.)

4. Meanwhile, for the slaw: In a small bowl, whisk together the vinegar, soy sauce, maple syrup, sesame oil, and ginger. In a large bowl, combine the cabbage, carrot, bell pepper, scallion, and cilantro. Drizzle the dressing over the vegetables and toss to combine.

5. To serve: In a small bowl, stir together the mayonnaise and sriracha. Make 8 stacks of 2 lettuce leaves per stack. Top each with 2 pieces of tofu and some slaw. Drizzle with the sriracha mayonnaise. Sprinkle with the sesame seeds and serve.

## Crispy Berbere-Roasted Tofu and Vegetables

*V, GF, CC*

*Makes 4 servings*

FOR THE TOFU AND VEGETABLES
    1 14-ounce block extra-firm tofu
    2 tablespoons ghee, butter, or vegan butter
    2 tablespoons extra-virgin olive oil
    1 tablespoon berbere seasoning (Ethiopian spice blend)
    2 carrots, peeled and cut diagonally into ½-inch-thick slices
    2 cups cauliflower florets
    Sea salt and freshly ground black pepper

FOR THE PICKLED RED ONIONS
    2 small red onions, peeled, halved, and thinly sliced
    ½ cup apple cider vinegar
    1 teaspoon maple syrup or 3 to 4 drops liquid stevia

Pinch cayenne
½ teaspoon ground coriander
½ teaspoon sea salt

1. For the tofu and vegetables: Preheat the oven to 400°F. Line a plate with two layers of paper towels. Place the tofu on the paper towels. Top with two additional layers of paper towels. Set a heavy skillet on top of the tofu and let stand for 15 minutes to press and drain off excess liquid. Cut the tofu into ¾-inch cubes. Place the tofu in a medium bowl and set aside.

2. In a small bowl, combine the melted butter, olive oil, and berbere seasoning. Stir well to combine. Place the carrots and cauliflower in a medium bowl. Drizzle about half of the berbere mixture over the tofu and the remaining half over the vegetables. Season both to taste with salt and pepper and toss each well to coat.

3. Arrange the tofu in a single layer on one side of a large rimmed baking sheet. Arrange the vegetables in a single layer on the other side of the pan. Roast until the tofu is golden brown and crispy and the vegetables are caramelized and beginning to brown, about 25 to 30 minutes, stirring once.

4. Meanwhile, for the pickled red onions: Place the onion in a small shallow heatproof bowl. In a small saucepan, combine the vinegar, maple syrup, cayenne, coriander, and salt. Bring to a boil. Pour over the onions, making sure they're completely submerged. Let stand 20 minutes. Drain the onions, reserving the brine for drizzling, if desired.

5. Divide the tofu and vegetables among 4 plates. Top the vegetables with the pickled onions and drizzle with some brine, if desired.

## Curried Tofu Scramble with Spinach and Tomatoes

*V, GF, CC*

*Makes 2 servings*

8 ounces extra-firm tofu
1 tablespoon ghee, butter, or vegan butter
2 tablespoons finely chopped red onion

½ cup cherry or grape tomatoes, halved
1 clove garlic, minced
1 5-ounce package baby spinach
½ to ¾ teaspoon curry powder
Sea salt and freshly ground black pepper
Whole-grain bread or naan, toasted (optional)

1. Line a plate with two layers of paper towels. Place the tofu on the paper towels. Top with two additional layers of paper towels. Set a heavy skillet on top of the tofu and let stand for 15 minutes to press and drain off excess liquid. Crumble the tofu and set aside.
2. In a medium nonstick skillet, heat the ghee over medium heat. Add the red onion and cook, stirring occasionally, for 2 to 3 minutes. Add the tomatoes and garlic and cook, stirring frequently, for an additional 2 to 3 minutes.
3. Reduce the heat to medium-low and add the spinach, tofu, and curry powder. Stir well to combine. Cover and cook for 4 to 5 minutes, stirring occasionally.
4. Season to taste with salt and pepper.
5. Serve with toasted bread or naan, if desired.

## Roasted Tempeh and Broccoli with Peanut Sauce

*V, GF, HT*

*Makes 2 servings*

FOR THE TEMPEH
    2 tablespoons low-sodium soy sauce or tamari
    1½ teaspoons pure maple syrup or 8 drops liquid stevia
    1 tablespoon sesame oil
    1 clove garlic, minced
    ¼ teaspoon red pepper flakes
    1 8-ounce package tempeh, cut into cubes or triangles

PEANUT SAUCE
    1 1-inch piece fresh ginger, peeled
    1 small clove garlic

½ cup natural creamy peanut butter

2 tablespoons low-sodium soy sauce or tamari

1 tablespoon fresh lime juice

1 teaspoon brown sugar or 5 drops liquid stevia

¼ to ½ teaspoon red pepper flakes

FOR THE BROCCOLI

1 small head broccoli, cut into florets

1 tablespoon sesame oil

Sea salt

Sesame seeds

1. For the tempeh: Preheat the oven to 425°F. Line two rimmed baking sheets with parchment paper or aluminum foil.

2. In a medium bowl, whisk together the soy sauce, maple syrup, sesame oil, garlic, and red pepper flakes. Add the tempeh and toss to coat. Marinate at room temperature for 20 minutes, stirring every 5 minutes.

3. Meanwhile, for the peanut sauce: With the motor running, drop the ginger and garlic into a blender and blend until finely chopped. Add the peanut butter, soy sauce, lime juice, brown sugar, red pepper flakes, and ⅓ cup water and blend, adding more water 1 tablespoon at a time if needed, until smooth and of pourable consistency. Set aside.

4. For the broccoli: In a large bowl, toss the broccoli florets with the sesame oil and salt to taste. Spread the broccoli florets on one of the prepared baking pans. Spread the marinated tempeh on the other prepared pan. Roast both the tempeh and broccoli for about 20 minutes, stirring each pan once. Remove the tempeh pan from the oven. Toss the tempeh with 2 tablespoons of the peanut sauce and return the tempeh pan to the oven. Roast the tempeh and the broccoli for another 5 minutes, or until the tempeh is browned and crisp and the broccoli is crisp-tender and lightly browned in spots.

5. Divide the tempeh and the broccoli between 2 plates. Drizzle with the remaining peanut sauce and sprinkle with sesame seeds.

# Spiced Moroccan Lentils

*V, GF, HT*

*Makes 4 servings*

### FOR THE RAS AL HANOUT SPICE MIX
½ teaspoon ground cumin
½ teaspoon ground ginger
1 teaspoon sea salt
½ freshly ground black pepper
¼ teaspoon ground cinnamon
¼ to ½ teaspoon cayenne
¼ teaspoon ground allspice
⅛ teaspoon ground cloves

### FOR THE LENTILS
¼ cup extra-virgin olive oil
½ teaspoon whole cumin seeds
½ teaspoon whole coriander seeds
1 small yellow onion, diced
4 cloves garlic, minced
1 cup crushed tomatoes
2 to 2½ cups water
1 cup whole brown or green lentils, rinsed
Finely grated zest of 1 lemon
2 tablespoons fresh lemon juice, plus more to taste
¼ cup minced freshly parsley
¼ cup minced fresh cilantro

### FOR SERVING
Hot cooked whole-grain couscous
Greek yogurt or plant-based yogurt

1. For the spice mix: In small bowl, stir together the cumin, ginger, salt, pepper, cinnamon, cayenne, allspice, and ground cloves. Set aside.
2. For the lentils: In a large saucepan, heat the olive oil over medium-high heat. When shimmering, add the cumin and coriander seeds. Allow to sizzle for 10 to 15 seconds or until

fragrant. Add the onion and cook, stirring frequently, until the onion is translucent and turning golden in spots. Add the garlic and cook until fragrant, about 15 seconds.

3. Add the spice mix to the pan and stir to coat everything in the oil and spices. Stir in the tomatoes and turn the heat to medium-low. Let simmer for 3 to 5 minutes until oil begins to pool on the surface. (This is called blooming the spices, which brings out their flavor.)

4. Add the water, starting with 2 cups, and the lentils. Bring to a boil. Reduce the heat to low, cover, and simmer until the lentils are tender but not mushy, about 30 to 40 minutes, stirring occasionally. Stir in the lemon zest. If the lentils look dry, add additional water.

5. When the lentils are the desired consistency, stir in the 2 tablespoons of lemon juice, parsley, and cilantro, adding more lemon juice, if desired.

6. To serve, ladle the lentils over hot cooked couscous and top with yogurt.

## SIDE DISHES, SOUPS, AND SALADS

### Brussels Sprouts Stir-Fry with Walnuts and Lemon

*V, GF, HT*

*Makes 4 servings*

2 tablespoons extra-virgin olive oil
1 pound Brussels sprouts, trimmed and thinly sliced
½ lemon
2 teaspoons walnut oil or sesame oil
Sea salt and freshly ground black pepper
⅓ cup coarsely chopped walnuts, toasted

1. In a large skillet, heat the olive oil over medium-high heat. Add the Brussels sprouts and cook, stirring frequently, until wilted and crisp-tender, about 5 to 6 minutes. (They should still be bright green.)

2. Remove from the heat. Finely grate the lemon over the sprouts, then squeeze the juice over. Drizzle with the walnut oil and season to taste with salt and pepper. Toss to combine. Scatter the walnuts over the sprouts and serve.

Variation: Pan-Seared Salmon with Lemon-Garlic Butter. To turn the Brussels Sprouts Stir-Fry with Walnuts and Lemon into a main dish, prepare that recipe through the first step. While the sprouts are cooking, pat dry 4 5- to 6-ounce salmon fillets. Season to taste with salt and pepper. Heat 1 tablespoon extra-virgin olive oil in a large nonstick skillet over medium-high heat. Place the fillets flesh side down in the pan, pressing lightly. Sear, undisturbed, for 3 to 4 minutes, until crispy and golden. Turn and sear the skin side for 2 minutes. Add 2 tablespoons butter; 2 cloves minced garlic; 3 tablespoons chopped fresh parsley; and 3 tablespoons fresh lemon juice + ½ lemon, sliced, to the pan, stirring around fish. Cook the salmon an additional 1 to 2 minutes, or until desired doneness. (The butter may start to brown slightly—that's okay.) Reserve the garlic butter from the pan. Divide the Brussels sprouts stir-fry among 4 plates. Sprinkle with the walnuts. Top the stir-fry with a salmon fillet. Drizzle each with lemon-garlic butter and sprinkle with about a tablespoon of chopped fresh parsley.

## Garlicky Baby Bok Choy and Shiitake Mushroom Stir-Fry

*V, GF, HT*

*Makes 4 servings*

1 tablespoon sesame oil
2 cloves garlic, thinly sliced
2 teaspoons grated fresh ginger
2 scallions, sliced, white and green parts separated
4 ounces shiitake mushrooms, stems removed, caps sliced
1 pound baby bok choy, rinsed, ends trimmed, sliced crosswise into ¾-inch pieces
1 tablespoon low-sodium soy sauce or tamari

1. In a wok or large skillet, heat the sesame oil over medium-high heat. Add the garlic, ginger, and scallion whites and cook, stirring constantly, until fragrant, about 30 seconds. Add the mushrooms and cook and stir until just starting to wilt, about 1 to 2 minutes. Add the boy choy, soy sauce, and 2 tablespoons water and cover. Stir to combine. Cover and cook for 1 minute. Uncover and toss, then cover and cook until the bok choy is crisp-tender, about 2 to 3 more minutes.
2. Sprinkle with the scallion greens. Serve immediately.

Variation: Garlicky Baby Bok Choy and Shiitake Mushroom Stir-Fry with Shrimp: To turn Garlicky Baby Bok Choy and Shiitake Mushroom Stir-Fry into a main dish, increase the sesame oil to 2 tablespoons and add an additional 1 teaspoon soy sauce. Add 1 pound shelled and deveined medium shrimp or plant-based shrimp to the pan with the mushrooms.

## Kimchi

*GF, V, HT*

*Makes 4 cups*

1 medium head napa cabbage
3 tablespoons plus 4 teaspoons sea salt
½ cup coarsely shredded daikon radish
½ cup coarsely shredded carrot
¼ cup chopped scallions
2 tablespoons fish sauce or vegan fish sauce
1 to 2 tablespoons gochugaru (Korean red chili powder)
1 tablespoon grated fresh ginger
2 cloves garlic, minced
1 teaspoon granulated sugar or 2 to 4 drops liquid stevia
1 quart water

1. Remove any wilted outer leaves from the cabbage. Core and cut the cabbage into 2-inch pieces. Measure 12 cups cabbage into a large bowl. Toss with the 3 tablespoons salt and place in a large colander set over the large bowl. Let stand 2 to 3 hours or until wilted.

2. In another large bowl combine the daikon, carrot, scallions, fish sauce, gochugaru, ginger, garlic, and sugar. Rinse the cabbage and drain well. Add the cabbage to daikon mixture and toss to combine. Let stand 10 minutes.
3. Transfer the cabbage mixture to a large ceramic crock, glass container, or plastic food container. Place a clean plate that just fits inside the container onto the mixture and press it down. Let the container stand at room temperature 2 to 24 hours or chill 5 to 24 hours, tossing the cabbage and pressing down on the plate every hour until enough liquid is released to cover the cabbage by at least 1 inch. (If necessary, add brine made in a ratio of 1 cup water to 1 teaspoon sea salt to cover.)
4. Place a large resealable plastic bag filled with the quart water plus the 4 teaspoons sea salt over the plate to weight it down. Cover the container with a clean kitchen towel or loose-fitting lid. To ferment, let the container stand out of direct sunlight at room temperature for 2 to 3 days or chill for 3 to 6 days. The kimchi is ready when it's bubbling.
5. Transfer the kimchi to clean jars or airtight containers. Store in the refrigerator for up to 3 weeks.

Note: Be sure your hands and all of your utensils are very clean to avoid introducing bad bacteria to the fermentation process.

## Yogurt Ranch Veggie Dip

*V (if plant-based yogurt is used), GF, HT*
*Makes about 1 cup*

1 cup Greek yogurt or plant-based yogurt
4 teaspoons dried parsley flakes
½ teaspoon dried dill
½ teaspoon garlic powder
½ teaspoon onion powder
½ teaspoon dried onion flakes
¼ teaspoon coarsely ground black pepper
½ teaspoon sea salt
1 tablespoon buttermilk powder (optional)

1. In a small bowl, stir together the yogurt, parsley, dill, garlic powder, onion powder, onion flakes, black pepper, sea salt, and buttermilk powder. Cover and chill for 1 hour to allow the flavors to blend. Keeps in the refrigerator for up to one week.

## Leek, Cabbage, and Sweet Potato Soup

*V, GF, HT*

*Makes 4 servings*

3 tablespoons extra-virgin olive oil
3 tablespoons butter or vegan butter
3 medium leeks, white and light green parts, thinly sliced
   (see Note)
8 cups shredded cabbage
2 cloves garlic, finely chopped
2 medium sweet potatoes, peeled and diced
2 cups chicken or vegetable broth
Sea salt
2 sprigs fresh thyme or ½ teaspoon dried thyme
Freshly ground black pepper
Chopped fresh chives (optional)

1. In a large saucepan, heat the olive oil and butter over medium-high heat. Add the leeks and cook until soft and golden on the edges, about 5 to 7 minutes. Add the cabbage and garlic and cook, stirring occasionally, until the cabbage begins to caramelize, about 10 minutes.
2. Stir in the sweet potatoes, broth, 4 cups water, salt to taste, and thyme. Bring to a simmer and cook, partially covered, until the potatoes are very tender, about 45 minutes. Add more water, if necessary, to reach the desired consistency. Season with black pepper to taste.
3. Remove the thyme sprigs and ladle the soup into 4 bowls. Sprinkle with fresh chives, if using.

Note: Leeks can contain a lot of sand and grit. The best way to clean them is to cut in half horizontally, thinly slice, and then swish the slices in a few changes of cool water. Spin them dry in a salad spinner if you have one—or simply drain and pat dry with paper towels. You don't want to sauté wet leeks—they'll get soggy instead of caramelizing nicely.

Variation: Leek, Cabbage, and Sweet Potato Soup with Beef: To make a heartier version of the Leek, Cabbage, and Sweet Potato Soup, prepare that recipe as instructed. Then brush an 8-ounce sirloin with extra-virgin olive oil and season to taste with sea salt, freshly ground black pepper, and smoked paprika. Broil to medium-rare (15 to 17 minutes for a 1-inch-thick steak, 25 to 27 minutes for a 1½-inch-thick steak), turning once. Let stand for 5 to 7 minutes, then thinly slice the beef and stir into the soup.

## Creamy Broccoli-Cheese Soup

*GF, HT*

*Makes 2 to 3 servings*

> 2 tablespoons butter or vegan butter
> 1 medium yellow onion, chopped
> 3 cloves garlic, smashed and peeled
> ¼ teaspoon red pepper flakes (optional)
> Sea salt and freshly ground black pepper
> 1 pound fresh broccoli (1 large or 2 small heads)
> 1 medium russet potato, peeled and cut into 1- to 2-inch chunks
> 3 cups chicken broth or water
> 3 to 4 ounces grated sharp cheddar cheese or vegan
>   cheddar cheese
> Sour cream, Greek yogurt, or vegan sour cream
> Thinly sliced chives or scallions

1. In a large saucepan, melt the butter over medium-low heat. Add the onion, garlic, red pepper flakes, if using, ⅛ teaspoon salt, and black pepper to taste. Cook, stirring occasionally, until the onions start to turn golden, about 6 to 8 minutes.
2. Meanwhile, cut the broccoli florets from the stalks and set aside. Trim the bottoms of the broccoli stalks. Use a vegetable peeler to remove the tough outer skin from the stalks. Slice the stalks into 1-inch-thick pieces. Set aside.

3. Add the broccoli stalks and potato to the pan. Add the chicken broth and ½ teaspoon salt. Bring to a boil, then reduce the heat to low and cover. Cook until the broccoli stalks and potato chunks are tender, about 20 minutes. Meanwhile, chop the reserved broccoli florets into smaller pieces.
4. Add half of the florets to the pan and cook until just bright green, about 3 to 5 minutes. Remove the pan from the heat and let cool slightly. Working in batches, carefully blend some of the soup in a blender until smooth, returning each batch to the pan as you work. (Alternatively, use an immersion blender.)
5. Return the pan to medium heat and add the remaining florets. Cover and cook just until the florets are bright green and crisp-tender, about 4 to 6 minutes. Add the cheese and stir until melted. Taste and adjust the seasonings, if desired.
6. To serve, ladle the soup into bowls. Swirl in a spoonful of sour cream and sprinkle with sliced chives or scallions.

## BEVERAGES

### Coconut Kefir

*V, GF, HT*

*Makes about 1 quart*

> 2 13.5-ounce cans full-fat coconut milk
> 1 5-gram packet kefir starter

1. Pour each can of coconut milk into a 16-ounce glass jar. Add half of the kefir starter packet to each jar. Stir well with a nonmetal spoon or wooden chopsticks.
2. Place a square of parchment paper over each jar and cover with the lid. Shake gently. Set the jars in a warm place, such as the top of the refrigerator, and let ferment for 24 to 48 hours.
3. Store in the refrigerator for up to 3 weeks.

## Iced Oat Milk Chai

*V, GF, HT*

*Makes 1 serving*

> 1 cup oat milk
> 1 scoop AmyMD Chai Latte Powder or any chai spice blend
> 2 to 4 drops liquid stevia
> ½ cup ice, plus more for serving
> Ground cinnamon, for dusting

1. In a cocktail shaker, combine the oat milk, Chai Latte Powder, stevia, and ice. Vigorously shake until thoroughly cold and the latte powder is dissolved, 10 to 15 seconds.
2. Strain into a tall ice-filled glass. Dust with cinnamon and serve immediately.

## Vanilla Chai Protein Shake

*V, GF, CC*

*Makes 1 serving*

> 1 cup unsweetened plant-based milk
> 1 scoop AmyMD Chai Latte Powder, or any chai spice blend
> 1 scoop unsweetened plant-based vanilla protein powder
> ½ frozen banana, cut into chunks
> ½ cup ice

In a blender, combine the plant-based milk, Chai Latte Powder, protein powder, banana, and ice. Blend on high until desired consistency, 1 to 2 minutes. (If the shake is too thick, add a little more plant-based milk or water.)

## Peppermint-Mocha Sipper

*V, GF, CC*

*Makes 1 serving*

> ¾ cup oat milk
> 1 tablespoon unsweetened cocoa powder, plus more for dusting
> 12 to 18 drops liquid stevia
> ¾ cup espresso or strong-brewed coffee
> 1 drop peppermint oil
> ¼ teaspoon pure vanilla extract

1. In a small saucepan, whisk together the oat milk, 1 tablespoon cocoa powder, and stevia. Add the coffee, peppermint oil, and vanilla. Heat, stirring frequently, until steaming and bubbles begin to form around the edges of the pan.
2. Pour into a mug and dust with cocoa powder. Serve immediately.

## Sweet Cherry–Almond Butter Smoothie

*V, GF, HT*

*Makes 1 smoothie*

> ¾ cup plant-based milk
> ¾ cup frozen dark sweet cherries
> ½ cup plain Greek yogurt or plant-based yogurt
> 1 tablespoon almond butter
> 1 scoop unsweetened plant-based vanilla protein powder
> ½ cup ice

1. In a blender, combine the plant-based milk, cherries, yogurt, almond butter, protein powder, and ice. Blend until smooth.

# Kombucha

*V, GF, HT*

*Makes 8 (16-ounce) bottles*

    16 cups purified water
    6 tea bags (green, black, white, or a combination)
    1 cup granulated sugar
    1 to 2 cups starter liquid (see Notes)
    1 SCOBY (see Notes)
    Optional flavorings

1. In a medium saucepan, bring 4 cups of the water to boiling. Remove from the heat and add the tea bags. Steep 15 minutes, then remove the tea bags and discard. Stir in the sugar until dissolved.

2. Meanwhile, add the remaining 12 cups water to a wide-mouth 1-gallon glass container. Add the sweetened tea to the container. Check the temperature of the mixture—it should be no warmer than about 100°F. Add the starter liquid and stir to combine. Add the SCOBY.

3. Cover the container with a paper towel, paper napkin, or tightly woven cloth and secure with a rubber band. Place in a warm (75°F to 80°F) ventilated area out of direct sunlight. Let stand for 7 days. (The mother SCOBY may rise to the top, sink, or float sideways, and a new baby SCOBY will form on top.)

4. To taste the brew, slide a straw under the SCOBYs. When the kombucha is the right balance of sweet and sour for your taste, decant it. If not, re-cover and continue fermenting, tasting every 2 days.

5. To decant, use clean hands to transfer the SCOBYs to a tall glass container along with 1 to 2 cups of the kombucha (this will serve as the starter liquid for the next batch). If you're making another batch immediately, cover the container with a paper towel or tightly woven cloth and set aside. If not, cover with a lid and refrigerate for up to 1 month.

6. For flavored kombucha, add the desired flavoring to each of 8 16-ounce bottles. Ladle the kombucha into the bottles through

a funnel, filling nearly to the top. Secure the lids and place out of direct sunlight for 1 to 3 days, burping the bottles daily to release carbonation and prevent explosions.

7. Place the bottles in the refrigerator and chill for at least 4 hours. Strain the flavorings from the kombucha before drinking.

OPTIONAL FLAVORINGS

Raspberry-hibiscus: Add 1 tablespoon gently mashed raspberries and ½ teaspoon dried hibiscus petals.

Lavender: Add 1 teaspoon dried lavender flowers.

Turmeric-ginger: Add 1½ teaspoons grated fresh turmeric root and 2 teaspoons grated fresh ginger.

NOTES

- Do not use herbal teas.
- You can purchase a SCOBY (symbiotic culture of bacteria and yeast) online or at most whole-foods markets.
- The starter liquid can be the liquid that comes with a purchased SCOBY or purchased plain kombucha.
- Finished kombucha will keep in the refrigerator for up to 3 weeks.

## TREATS

## Dark Chocolate–Dipped Fruit

*V, GF, CC*

*Makes 24 pieces*

8 ounces sugar-free dark chocolate chips or sugar-free vegan chocolate chips

8 dried apricots

8 pieces dried apple

8 dried plums (prunes)

Sea salt, flaked variety

Pistachios, almonds, and/or walnuts, toasted and finely chopped (see Note)

1. Line a large rimmed baking sheet with parchment paper.
2. In a medium microwave-safe bowl, microwave the chocolate chips at 50% power in 30-second intervals, stirring after each interval, until smooth. Set aside to cool slightly, about 5 minutes.
3. Dip the apricots, apples, and plums in the chocolate and place on the prepared baking sheet. Sprinkle with flaky salt or chopped nuts immediately.
4. When all of the fruit is coated and sprinkled, place the baking sheet in the refrigerator to allow the chocolate to set.
5. Store in the refrigerator in a tightly sealed container for up to one week. For the best taste and texture, allow to come to room temperature before serving.

Note: You can use all of one kind of nut—or none at all—but pistachios pair particularly well with apricots, walnuts with apples, and almonds with dried plums. You can also make just one or two kinds of fruits—whatever you prefer.

## Dark Chocolate–Peppermint Coins with Cacao Nibs

*V, GF, CC*

*Makes about 40 pieces*

8 ounces sugar-free dark chocolate chips or sugar-free vegan chocolate chips
2 drops peppermint oil
½ cup cacao nibs

1. Line a large rimmed baking sheet with parchment paper.
2. In a medium microwave-safe bowl, microwave the chocolate chips at 50% power in 30-second intervals, stirring after each interval, until smooth.
3. Drop tablespoon-size spoonfuls of the chocolate at least 2 inches apart on the prepared pan. Bang the pan on the counter once or twice to spread the chocolate into thin pools about 2 inches wide.

4. Immediately, while the chocolate is still liquid, sprinkle each with a generous ½ teaspoon cacao nibs. Place the baking sheet in the refrigerator to allow the chocolate to set.
5. Store in the refrigerator in a tightly sealed container for up to one week. For the best taste and texture, allow to come to room temperature before serving.

## Fudgy Black Bean Brownies

*V, GF, HT, CC*

*Makes 9 brownies*

> 1 15-ounce can black beans, drained and rinsed
> 2 tablespoons unsweetened cocoa powder
> ½ cup quick oats
> ¼ teaspoon sea salt
> ½ cup maple pure maple syrup or 1 teaspoon liquid stevia
> ¼ cup coconut oil, plus more for greasing the pan
> 2 teaspoons pure vanilla extract
> 1 teaspoon instant espresso powder
> ½ cup sugar-free dark chocolate chips or sugar-free vegan chocolate chips

1. Preheat the oven to 350°F. Grease an 8x8-inch baking pan with some coconut oil.
2. In a food processor, combine the beans, cocoa powder, oats, salt, maple syrup, ¼ cup coconut oil, vanilla extract, and espresso powder. Blend until completely smooth. Stir in the chocolate chips.
3. Pour the batter into the prepared pan. Bake 15 to 18 minutes, or until the surface looks mostly dry but is still a little glossy.
4. Cool in the pan on a wire rack for at least 10 minutes before cutting. (If the brownies still look a little bit undercooked, chill in the refrigerator overnight before cutting.)

## Pumpkin Spice Chia Seed Pudding

*V, GF, CC*

*Makes 4 servings*

2¼ cups unsweetened plant-based milk
1 cup pumpkin puree
2 tablespoons pure maple syrup or ¼ teaspoon liquid stevia
½ teaspoon pure vanilla extract
5 tablespoons chia seeds
2 teaspoons pumpkin pie spice
Pinch sea salt
¼ cup pecans
2 tablespoons pepita seeds

1. In a medium bowl, whisk together the plant-based milk, pumpkin puree, maple syrup, vanilla extract, and chia seeds. Add the pumpkin pie spice and salt and whisk to combine. Cover and refrigerate until thick and pudding-like, about 2 to 3 hours.
2. To serve, spoon the pudding into 4 bowls or dishes. Top with the pecans and pepita seeds.

Note: The pudding can be made in advance and stored in an airtight container in the refrigerator for up to 4 days.

## Green Tea Yogurt Bowl with Berries and Chocolate

*GF, V (if plant-based yogurt is used), HT, CC*

*Makes 1 serving*

¾ cup plain Greek yogurt or plant-based yogurt
1 scoop unsweetened plant-based vanilla protein powder
1 teaspoon high-quality matcha powder
½ to ¾ teaspoon agave or 3 to 5 drops liquid stevia
Fresh berries, such as raspberries, blueberries, or blackberries
1 tablespoon sugar-free dark chocolate chips

In a small bowl, whisk together the yogurt, protein powder, matcha powder, and agave until smooth. Top with fresh berries and the chocolate chips. Serve immediately.

# Acknowledgments

As the pandemic drags into 2022, my perspective on life has changed a little bit. After I wrote my last book, I thanked everyone—literally everyone on the planet that I could think of. Part of it was out of gratitude and part of it was out of fear that I would forget someone!

Well, now I don't have that fear anymore since I've already thanked everyone who needs to be thanked!

That's the crux of this book, too—no fear of what others would think of my opinions, and that's how I wrote it. I wanted it to be transparent, scientific, and, most of all, applicable.

As I do, I want you to live a fearless yet peaceful life. I want you to identify what you're really hungry for. This will give you freedom of mind and body—which is of the utmost importance.

I want to thank my parents, brother, friends, and family for putting up with me during this journey. Especially my darling husband, who first entertained my silly ideas and then realized that they were becoming a book and a business! Little did he know that he was going on this crazy journey with me. But I wouldn't have been able to do it without his support. I wish for every woman to find a partner with whom they feel free to grow. We are so blessed with two gems as children.

I want to thank my wonderful agent, Heather Jackson, who is not only my agent but also my guide through the publishing process. I want to thank my publisher, HarperCollins, and specifically Sarah Pelz—it's been a dream to work with someone who is so in tune with the health world and the book world at the same time. Thank you for giving me a chance to work with you again. Thank you to my collaborator, Maggie Greenwood-Robinson, for being so kind and patient with my texts, notes, and busy schedule.

The following quote from Bobby Flay via Tim Ferriss really sums up my last three years: "Take risks and you'll get the payoffs. Learn from your mistakes until you succeed. It's that simple."

I have failed but I have learned from my mistakes. Thank you for your interest in this book and most importantly thank you for your interest in science.

# Bibliography

## INTRODUCTION: IT'S NOT YOUR FAULT

American Diabetes Association. Statistics, www.diabetes.org.

Bermudez-Humaran, L. G., et al. 2019. From Probiotics to Psychobiotics: Live Beneficial Bacteria Which Act on the Brain-Gut Axis. *Nutrients* 11: 890.

Hallam, J., et al. 2016. Gender-related Differences in Food Craving and Obesity. *The Yale Journal of Biology and Medicine* 89: 161–173.

Lehto, S. A., et al. 2016. Psychobiotics and the Manipulation of Bacteria-Gut Brain Signals. *Trends in Neuroscience* 39: 763–781.

Thompson, M. 2019. Health and Fitness Industry Statistics. AXcess News, axcessnews.com/national/health/health-and-fitness-industry-statistics-2019-10771/.

## CHAPTER 1: HOW DID MY HUNGER GET SO EFFED UP?

Arterburn, L. M., et al. 2008. Algal-Oil Capsules and Cooked Salmon: Nutritionally Equivalent Sources of Docosahexaenoic Acid. *Journal of the American Dietetic Association* 108: 1204–1209.

Cork, S. C. 2018. The Role of the Vagus Nerve in Appetite Control: Implications for the Pathogenesis of Obesity. *Journal of Neuroendocrinology* 30: e12643.

Hall, K. D., et al. 2019. Ultra-Processed Diets Cause Excess Calorie Intake and Weight Gain: An Inpatient Randomized Controlled Trial of Ad Libitum Food Intake. *Cell Metabolism* 30: 67–77.

Huberman, A. 2021. *How Our Hormones Control Our Hunger, Eating &
Satiety*. Podcast, April 19, hubermanlab.com/how-our-hormones
-control-our-hunger-eating-and-satiety/.

Kozimor, A., et al. 2013. Effects of Dietary Fatty Acid Composition
from a High Fat Meal on Satiety. *Appetite* 69: 39–45.

Ravussin, E., et al. 2019. Early Time-Restricted Feeding Reduces
Appetite and Increases Fat Oxidation but Does Not Affect Energy
Expenditure in Humans. *Obesity* 27: 1244–1254.

Schroeder. J. 2013. Are Oreos Addictive? Research Says Yes. *Science
Daily*, October.

Sohn, J. 2015. Network of Hypothalamic Neurons that Control
Appetite. *BMB Reports* 48(4): 229–233.

Zagmutt, S., et al. 2018. Targeting AgRP Neurons to Maintain Energy
Balance: Lessons from Animal Models. *Biochemical Pharmacology*
155: 224–232.

Zanchi, D., et al. 2017. The Impact of Gut Hormones on the Neural
Circuit of Appetite and Satiety: A Systematic Review. *Neuroscience
and Biobehavioral Reviews* 80: 457–475.

## CHAPTER 2: THE HUNGER HIJACKERS

Akyol, A., et al. 2019. Impact of Three Different Plate Colours on
Short-term Satiety and Energy Intake: A Randomized Controlled
Trial. *The Nutrition Journal* 17: 46.

Bruno, N., et al. 2013. The Effect of the Color Red on Consuming
Food Does Not Depend on Achromatic (Michelson) Contrast
and Extends to Rubbing Cream on the Skin. *Appetite* 71:
307–313.

Johnson, J. 2018. Fad Diets Are Bad Diets. American Council on
Science and Health, www.acsh.org.

Lakhano, N., et al. 2021. American Council on Science and Health
Revealed: The True Extent of America's Food Monopolies, and
Who Pays the Price. *Guardian*, July.

Tomova, L., et al. 2020. Acute Social Isolation Evokes Midbrain
Craving Responses Similar to Hunger. *Nature Neuroscience* 23:
1597–1605.

Van Doorn, G. H., et al. 2014. Does the Colour of the Mug Influence the Taste of the Coffee? *Flavour* 3, November 25.

## CHAPTER 3: THE POWER OF PSYCHOBIOTICS

Abisado, R. G., et al. 2018. Bacterial Quorum Sensing and Microbial Community Interactions. *mBIO* 9: e02331-17.

Alcock, J., et al. 2014. Is Eating Behavior Manipulated by the Gastrointestinal Microbiota? Evolutionary Pressures and Potential Mechanisms. *Bioessays* 36: 940–949.

Crovesy, L., et al. 2020. Profile of the Gut Microbiota of Adults with Obesity: A Systematic Review. *European Journal of Clinical Nutrition* 74: 1251–1262.

Dinan, T. G., and Cryan, J.F. 2017. The Microbiome-Gut-Brain Axis in Health and Disease. *Gastroenterology Clinics of North America* 46: 77–89.

Jäger, R., et al. 2019. International Society of Sports Nutrition Position Stand: Probiotics. *International Society of Sports Nutrition* 16: 62.

Jacques, P. F., and Wang, H. 2014. Yogurt and Weight Management. *The American Journal of Clinical Nutrition* 99 (5 Supplement): 1229S–1234S.

Martin, F. P., et al. 2012. Specific Dietary Preferences Are Linked to Differing Gut Microbial Metabolic Activity in Response to Dark Chocolate Intake. *Journal of Proteome Research,* Epub, November.

Schmidt, K., et al. 2015. Prebiotic Intake Reduces the Waking Cortisol Response and Alters Emotional Bias in Healthy Volunteers. *Psychopharmacology* 232: 1793–1801.

Song, S. J., et al. 2013. Cohabiting Family Members Share Microbiota with One Another and with Their Dogs. *Elife* 2: e00458.

Steenbergen, L., et al. 2015. A Randomized Controlled Trial to Test the Effect of Multispecies Probiotics on Cognitive Reactivity to Sad Mood. *Brain, Behavior, and Immunity* 48: 258–264.

Xiang Ng, Q., et al. 2018. A Meta-Analysis of the Use of Probiotics to Alleviate Depressive Symptoms. *Journal of Affective Disorders* 228: 13–19.

Yoona, K., et al. 2016. Polyphenols and Glycemic Control. *Nutrients* 8: 17.

Zheng, P., et al. 2019. The Gut Microbiome from Patients with Schizophrenia Modulates the Glutamate-Glutamine-GABA Cycle and Schizophrenia-Relevant Behaviors in Mice. *Science Advances* 5: eaau8317.

## CHAPTER 4: UNLEARNED EATING

Sakkas, H., et al. 2020. Nutritional Status and the Influence of the Vegan Diet on the Gut Microbiota and Human Health. *Medicina* 56: 88.

Wise, P. M., et al. 2016. Reduced Dietary Intake of Simple Sugars Alters Perceived Sweet Taste Intensity but Not Perceived Pleasantness. *The American Journal of Clinical Nutrition* 103: 50–60.

## CHAPTER 5: STEP 1: REPLENISH

Anderson, J. W., et al. 2019. Health Benefits of Dietary Fiber. *Nutrition Reviews* 67: 188–205.

Farr, O. M., et al. 2018. Walnut Consumption Increases Activation of the Insula to Highly Desirable Food Cues: A Randomized, Double-Blind, Placebo-Controlled, Cross-Over fMRI Study. *Diabetes, Obesity, and Metabolism* 20: 173–177.

Gray, B., et al. 2013. Omega-3 Fatty Acids: A Review of the Effects on Adiponectin and Leptin and Potential Implications for Obesity Management. *European Journal of Clinical Nutrition* 6: 1234–1242.

Hiel, S., et al. 2019. Effects of a Diet Based on Inulin-Rich Vegetables on Gut Health and Nutritional Behavior in Healthy Humans. *The American Journal of Clinical Nutrition* 109: 1683–1695.

Lazutkaite, G., et al. 2017. Amino Acid Sensing in Hypothalamic Tanycytes via Umami Taste Receptors. *Molecular Metabolism* 6: 1480–1492.

Leri, M., et al. 2020. Healthy Effects of Plant Polyphenols: Molecular Mechanisms. *International Journal of Molecular Sciences* 21: 1250.

Ortinau, L. C., et al. 2014. Effects of High-Protein vs. High-Fat Snacks on Appetite Control, Satiety, and Eating Initiation in Healthy Women. *Nutrition Journal* 13: 97.

Parra, D., et al. 2008. A Diet Rich in Long Chain Omega-3 Fatty Acids Modulates Satiety in Overweight and Obese Volunteers during Weight Loss. *Appetite* 51: 676–680.

Prieto, M. A., et al. 2019. Glucosinolates: Molecular Structure, Breakdown, Genetic, Bioavailability, Properties and Healthy and Adverse Effects. *Advances in Food and Nutrition Research* 90: 305–350.

Reed, J. A., et al. 2008. Effects of Peppermint Scent on Appetite Control and Caloric Intake. *Appetite* 51: 393.

Rigamonti, A., et al. 2020. The Appetite-Suppressant and GLP-1-Stimulating Effects of Whey Proteins in Obese Subjects Are Associated with Increased Circulating Levels of Specific Amino Acids. *Nutrients* 12: 775.

Roberfroid, M., et al. 2010. Prebiotic Effects: Metabolic and Health Benefits. *British Journal of Nutrition* 104 Supplement 2: S1–63.

Şanlier, N., et al. 2019. Health Benefits of Fermented Foods. *Critical Reviews in Food Science and Nutrition* 59: 506–527.

Tome, D., et al. 2009. Protein, Amino Acids, Vagus Nerve Signaling, and the Brain. *The American Journal of Clinical Nutrition* 90: 838S–843S.

Tremblay, A., et al. 2015. Impact of Yogurt on Appetite Control, Energy Balance, and Body Composition. *Nutrition Reviews* 73 Supplement 1: 23–27.

Wastyk, H., et al. 2021. Gut-Microbiota-Targeted Diets Modulate Human Immune Status. *Cell* 184: 4137–4153.

Zemel, M., and Bruckbauer, A. 2013. Effects of a Leucine and Pyridoxine-Containing Nutraceutical on Body Weight and Composition in Obese Subjects. *Diabetes, Metabolic Syndrome, and Obesity: Targets and Therapy* 6: 309–315.

CHAPTER 6: STEP 2: REWIRE

Deckersbach, T., et al. 2014. Pilot Randomized Trial Demonstrating Reversal of Obesity-Related Abnormalities in Reward System Responsivity to Food Cues with a Behavioral Intervention. *Nutrition & Diabetes* 4: e129.

Goodridge, A., et al. 2013. Food Addiction: Its Prevalence and Significant Association with Obesity in the General Population. *PLOS One* 8: e74832.

Guiliani, N., et al. 2013. Piece of Cake: Cognitive Reappraisal of Food Craving. *Appetite* 64: 56–61.

Huberman, A. 2021. How to Increase Motivation and Drive. March 22, hubermanlab.com./how-to-increase-motivation-and-drive/.

Kuijer, R. G., et al. 2014. Chocolate Cake: Guilt or Celebration? Associations with Healthy Eating Attitudes, Perceived Behavioural Control, Intentions and Weight-Loss. *Appetite* 74: 48–54.

Patrick, V. M., and Hagtvedt, H. 2012. "I Don't" versus "I Can't": When Empowered Refusal Motivates Goal-Directed Behavior. *Journal of Consumer Research* 39: 371–381.

Strachan, S. M., and Brawley, L.R. 2009. Healthy-Eater Identity and Self-Efficacy Predict Healthy Eating Behavior: A Prospective View. *Journal of Health Psychology* 14: 684–695.

## CHAPTER 7: STEP 3: RESET

American Psychological Association. 2020. Stress in America 2020: A National Mental Health Crisis.

Cedernaes, J., et al. 2019. Transcriptional Basis for Rhythmic Control of Hunger and Metabolism within the AgRP Neuron. *Cell Metabolism* 29: 1078–1091.

Davis, N., and Sample, I. 2017. Nobel Prize for Medicine Awarded for Insights into Internal Biological Clock. *Guardian*, October 2.

Huang, W., et al. 2011. Circadian Rhythms, Sleep, and Metabolism. *The Journal of Clinical Investigation* 121: 2133–2141.

Law, R., et al. 2020. Stress, the Cortisol Awakening Response and Cognitive Function. *International Review of Neurobiology* 150: 187–217.

Longo, V. D., and Panda, S. et al. 2016. Fasting, Circadian Rhythms, and Time-Restricted Feeding in Healthy Lifespan. *Cell Metabolism* 23: 1048–1059.

Pot, G. K., et al. 2016. Meal Irregularity and Cardiometabolic Consequences: Results from Observational and Intervention Studies. *Proceedings of the Nutrition Society* 75: 475–486.

Ravussin, E., et al. 2019. Early Time-Restricted Feeding Reduces Appetite and Increases Fat Oxidation but Does Not Affect Energy Expenditure in Humans. *Obesity* 27: 1244–1254.

Russell, G., and Lightman, S. 2019. The Human Stress Response. *Nature Reviews—Endocrinology* 15: 525–534.

Turekcorinne, F. W., et al. 2005. Obesity and Metabolic Syndrome in Circadian Clock Mutant Mice. *Science* 308: 1043–1045.

## CHAPTER 8: STEP 4: REFRESH

Beil, L. 2021. How Sleep Affects Your Blood Sugar. WebMD.com, July 25, https://www.webmd.com/diabetes/sleep-affects-blood-sugar.

Broussard, J. L., et al. 2016. Elevated Ghrelin Predicts Food Intake During Experimental Sleep Restriction. *Obesity* 24: 132–138.

Cappuccio, F., et al. 2010. Sleep Duration and All-Cause Mortality: a Systematic Review and Meta-Analysis of Prospective Studies. *Sleep* 33: 585–592.

Henst, R. H. P., et al. 2019. The Effects of Sleep Extension on Cardiometabolic Risk Factors: A Systematic Review. *Journal of Sleep Research* 28: e12865.

Katano, S., et al. 2011. Association of Short Sleep Duration with Impaired Glucose Tolerance or Diabetes Mellitus. *Journal of Diabetes Investigation* 2: 366–372.

Owens, B. 2013. Obesity: Heavy Sleepers. *Nature* 497: S8–S9 (2013).

St. Onge, M. P., et al. 2016. Fiber and Saturated Fat Are Associated with Sleep Arousals and Slow Wave Sleep. *Journal of Clinical Sleep Medicine* 12: 19–24.

Suni, E. 2021. Sleep Deprivation. National Sleep Foundation, June 24, https://www.sleepfoundation.org/sleep-deprivation.

Underner, M., et al. 2006. Cigarette Smoking and Sleep Disturbance. *La Revue des Maladies Respiratoires* 23 (3 Supplement): 6S67–6S77.

Allen, J. M., et al. 2018. Exercise Alters Gut Microbiota Composition and Function in Lean and Obese Humans. *Medicine and Science in Sports and Exercise* 50: 747–757.

Berman, M. G., et al. 2008. The Cognitive Benefits of Interacting with Nature. *Psychological Science* 19: 1207–1212.

Broom, D. R. 2009. Influence of Resistance and Aerobic Exercise on Hunger, Circulating Levels of Acylated Ghrelin, and Peptide YY in Healthy Males. *American Journal of Physiology—Regulatory, Integrative and Comparative Physiology* 296: R29–R35.

Fillon, A., et al. 2020. Appetite Control and Exercise: Does the Timing of Exercise Play a Role? *Physiology and Behavior* 218: 112733.

Freitas, M. C., et al. 2019. Appetite Is Suppressed After Full-Body Resistance Exercise Compared with Split-Body Resistance Exercise: The Potential Influence of Lactate and Autonomic Modulation. *Journal of Strength and Conditioning Research,* 35: 2532–2540.

Larson-Meyer, D. E., et al. 2012. Influence of Running and Walking on Hormonal Regulators of Appetite in Women. *Journal of Obesity,* April 29.

Lim, S. A., and Cheong, K. J. 2015. Regular Yoga Practice Improves Antioxidant Status, Immune Function, and Stress Hormone Releases in Young Healthy People: A Randomized, Double-Blind, Controlled Pilot Study. *Journal of Complementary and Alternative Medicine* 21: 530–538.

McIver, S., et al. 2009. Yoga as a Treatment for Binge Eating Disorder: A Preliminary Study. *Complementary Therapies in Medicine* 17: 196–202.

Watts, A. W., et al. 2018. Yoga's Potential for Promoting Healthy Eating and Physical Activity Behaviors Among Young Adults. *International Journal of Behavioral Nutrition and Physical Activity* 15: 42.

Young, S. N. 2007. How to Increase Serotonin in the Human Brain without Drugs. *Journal of Psychiatry and Neuroscience* 32: 394–399.

# Index

modifying food memories, 63–65
recognizing true hunger vs. boredom, 65
tuning into bodyset, 69–70

vagus nerve, 6–7, 20
Vanilla Chai Protein Shake, 197
vegetables, 3, 19, 133. *See also specific vegetables*
fiber in, 53–54, 67–68, 68, 86–88
glucosinolates in, 77–78
high in water, 68–69
nutrient density of, 57
polyphenols in, 79
Raw Veggie Test, 70–71
shopping lists, 164–65, 167–68
vegetarian diet, xiii, xv, 3, 17
vinegar, 55
vitamin B1 (thiamine), 41
vitamin B2 (riboflavin), 41
vitamin B6, 12, 83
vitamin B12, 41
vitamin D, 7, 12, 146
vitamin K2, 41

walnuts, 85, 86, 89–90, 91, 166, 169
weight gain, xii, xv–xvi, 19, 24, 84, 117

weight loss
adjusting eating behavior little at a time, 102–3
author's father's story, xiv
Cyndie's story, xxi–xxii
diet industry, xii, xxi–xxii, 24, 34–36, 39
gut microbiome and, 42, 43
Marcy's story, 59–60
Monica's story, x–xi
Robert's story, 38–39
Western model of medicine, xvi
white flour, 29–30
white sugar, 30
whole foods, 16, 17, 19
whole grains, 3, 19, 53, 68, 91
willpower, xi, 35, 39, 59, 60, 62, 69, 76, 129, 146
workouts. *See* exercise

Yale Food Addiction Scale, 94–95
yoga, xviii, xxv, 27, 119, 143–44, 147, 149, 152
yogurt, 43, 52, 56, 76, 88–89, 91, 158
recipes, 177–79, 193–94, 203
Yogurt Ranch Veggie Dip, 193–94
Young, Michael W., 112

# About the Author

Dr. Amy Shah has one of the most unique training backgrounds in the world. She trained at the renowned school of nutrition at Cornell University, where she graduated magna cum laude, and then she went on to graduate from medical school with honors for her research in her publication "CT Detection of Acute Myocardial Infarction."

After obtaining expertise in both nutrition and medicine at Albert Einstein College of Medicine, Dr. Shah then completed her residency and fellowship at Harvard Medical School's teaching hospital Beth Israel Deaconess Medical Center and at Columbia University hospitals, respectively.

In addition to her clinical work, she wrote her first book in 2021, called *I'm So Effing Tired*.

Dr. Shah frequently speaks to companies and events, including Morgan Stanley, Goldman Sachs, Brave Enough Women's CME Conference, NBC Universal, Women in Retail Leadership Summit, and TPG. She has been a guest on top local and national television shows such as KTLA Morning News and the *Today* show and podcasts like *The Genius Life, The Dr. Axe Show, Bulletproof Radio,* and many more.

Dr. Shah loves to innovate in the wellness and nutrition world. Her website is amymdwellness.com.